MEAT PUPPETS: HOW PARASITES CONTROL YOUR BODY, MIND & SPIRIT

Other Works By This Author:

WEAPONS GRADE MOXIE: UNLEASHING YOUR INNER STRENGTH TO CONQUER FEAR AND TOXIC PEOPLE

YOU ARE INFINITE!: CO-CREATING THE FRACTAL HOLOGRAPH

UNSTUCK: EXPERIENCING THE ANAHATA NAD

THE PINEAL PORTAL: UNLOCKING THE SECRETS OF THE THIRD EYE

LIFE IN THE BLISS LANE: A GUIDE TO WELLNESS, SELF-LOVE, AND JOY

KILLING TIME: BREAKING FREE FROM TEMPORAL CHAINS

LEVEL UP WITH GRATITUDE: THE ULTIMATE BIO-HACK FOR HAPPINESS

ARDHANARISHWARA CHARITRA: THE METAPHYSICAL WISDOM OF GENDER FLUIDITY

VASUDHAIVA KUTUMBAKAM: THE LIMITLESS POWER OF OUR DESI ROOTS

THE ATMA'S JOURNEY: TAROT WISDOM THROUGH THE RAMAYANA & MAHABHARATA

YOU MAKE ME SICK: VIRTUE SIGNALING & NARCISSISTIC ABUSE

TOXIC SIBLING ESTRANGEMENT: RECLAIMING YOUR INNER PEACE

HIDDEN BRANCHES IN THE FAMILY TREE: NAVIGATING THE NPE EXPERIENCE

BEYOND BINARY: AN EXPLORATION IN GENDER AND SEXUALITY

PHARMAJUANA: GUIDE TO CANNABIS FOR CANCER

WHY STRAIGHT LINES DON'T EXIST: EXPLORING GEOMETRIC TRUTHS

HOW TO GYM: BECOMING FITNESS ITSELF

MEAT PUPPETS: HOW PARASITES CONTROL YOUR BODY, MIND & SPIRIT

MEAT PUPPETS: HOW PARASITES CONTROL YOUR BODY, MIND & SPIRIT

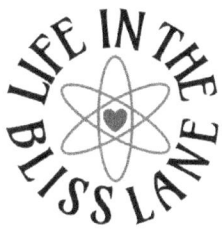

@2024

Life in the Bliss Lane

Dr. Sunayana Shivangi Pandé

MEAT PUPPETS: HOW PARASITES CONTROL YOUR BODY, MIND & SPIRIT

For Yogi

THE FIRST PARASITE I KNEW INTIMATELY

MEAT PUPPETS: HOW PARASITES CONTROL YOUR BODY, MIND & SPIRIT

TABLE OF CONTENTS

PART 1 1

The Hidden Influence of Parasites on Our Lives 2

DEFINING PARASITES: BIOLOGICAL AND SPIRITUAL PERSPECTIVES 3
ANCIENT WISDOM: THE INDIAN PERSPECTIVE ON PARASITES 4
THE CONSUMPTION OF MEAT: A GATEWAY TO PARASITIC INFLUENCE ... 5
RECLAIMING CONTROL OVER OUR HEALTH AND SPIRITUALITY 6

PART 2 8

The Ayurvedic Perspective on Parasites 9

UNDERSTANDING KRIMI VIDYA: THE SCIENCE OF PARASITES 9
AYURVEDIC TREATMENTS FOR PARASITIC INFESTATIONS 12
SPIRITUAL AND PHYSICAL INTERCONNECTEDNESS 15

Parasites in Hindu Mythology and Practices 18

MYTHOLOGICAL REFERENCES: THE PARASITIC INFLUENCE IN HINDU LORE . 18
CONNECTING MYTHOLOGICAL REFERENCES TO PHYSICAL REALITY 21
HINDU PRACTICES FOR PROTECTION 23

PART 3 28

Cats in Hinduism, Ayurveda, and Parasitology 29

CATS AS SPIRITUAL ENTITIES IN HINDUISM 29
THE AYURVEDIC VIEW ON CATS 31
TOXOPLASMA GONDII AND THE SPIRITUAL CONNECTION 34
CATS, PARASITES, AND THE SPIRITUAL DIMENSION 37

The Biblical and Cultural Views of Parasites 41

BIBLICAL PERSPECTIVES ON PARASITES AS DEMONIC INFLUENCES 41
THE REMOVAL OF FASTING FROM THE BIBLE: SPIRITUAL AND PHYSICAL CONSEQUENCES 45
CULTURAL BELIEFS ABOUT PARASITES AND THEIR SPIRITUAL SIGNIFICANCE 47
THE SATTVIK LIFESTYLE: MINIMIZING EXPOSURE TO PARASITES 50

PART 4 54

How Parasites Manipulate Human Behavior 55
- TOXOPLASMA GONDII AND BEHAVIORAL CHANGES 55
- OTHER COMMON PARASITES AND THEIR IMPACT ON HUMAN BEHAVIOR 58
- THE BROADER IMPLICATIONS OF PARASITIC INFLUENCE ON MENTAL AND SPIRITUAL HEALTH 62
- PARASITES AND SUICIDAL IDEATION: THE HIDDEN INFLUENCE ON MENTAL HEALTH 64
- THE SOCIAL AND CULTURAL IMPLICATIONS 67

Parasites, Demons, and the Weakening of Spiritual Sovereignty 70
- THE SPIRITUAL AND PHYSICAL CONSEQUENCES OF PARASITIC INFECTION . 70
- AYURVEDIC AND HINDU SOLUTIONS FOR RECLAIMING SPIRITUAL SOVEREIGNTY 73
- THE ROLE OF FASTING IN MAINTAINING SPIRITUAL SOVEREIGNTY 77

PART 5 82

Ayurvedic Detoxification and Fasting 83
- THE ROLE OF PANCHAKARMA IN CLEANSING PARASITES 83
- FASTING IN HINDUISM AND AYURVEDA 86
- INCORPORATING SALT AND HERBS IN DETOXIFICATION 89
- THE INTEGRATION OF FASTING AND DETOXIFICATION INTO MODERN LIFE ... 92

Reclaiming Spiritual Sovereignty Through Hindu Practices 96
- SPIRITUAL PRACTICES FOR PROTECTION 96
- THE POWER OF MANTRAS AND RITUALS 101
- RECLAIMING SPIRITUAL SOVEREIGNTY THROUGH HINDU PRACTICES 103

Integrating Ayurveda and Hinduism in Modern Life 107
- DAILY PRACTICES FOR HEALTH AND SPIRITUALITY 107
- THE CULTURAL SHIFT: MOVING BEYOND MEAT CONSUMPTION 111
- INTEGRATING SPIRITUAL PRACTICES IN DAILY LIFE 114
- THE PATH FORWARD: EMBRACING A HOLISTIC APPROACH 117

CONCLUSION: 121

The Path to Liberation 122

SYNTHESIS OF AYURVEDIC AND HINDU WISDOM 122
A CALL TO ACTION: EMBRACE THE PATH TO LIBERATION 125
FINAL REFLECTIONS 127

ABOUT THE AUTHOR 129

PART 1

INTRODUCTION

In the modern world, we often think of parasites as mere nuisances—unpleasant but ultimately manageable threats to our health. We might associate them with poor sanitation, tropical climates, or undercooked food, but rarely do we consider the profound impact they have on our bodies, minds, and spirits. However, what if I told you that parasites are more than just biological organisms? What if these seemingly simple creatures could influence your thoughts, behaviors, and even your spiritual well-being?

THE HIDDEN INFLUENCE OF PARASITES ON OUR LIVES

This book explores a startling and often overlooked aspect of human life—the way in which parasites, particularly those contracted through meat consumption, can compromise our autonomy and spiritual health. By viewing parasites through the lenses of Ayurveda, Hinduism, and ancient wisdom, we will uncover the ways in which these microscopic invaders parallel the demonic forces described in religious and spiritual traditions.

MEAT PUPPETS: HOW PARASITES CONTROL YOUR BODY, MIND & SPIRIT

DEFINING PARASITES: BIOLOGICAL AND SPIRITUAL PERSPECTIVES

Parasites, in the simplest biological terms, are organisms that live at the expense of their host. They survive by feeding on the host's resources, often causing harm in the process. But parasites are more than just physical entities; they are manifestations of deeper imbalances in our lives—imbalances that can affect not just our bodies, but our minds and spirits as well.

In Ayurveda, the ancient Indian system of medicine, parasites are understood as *krimi*—foreign invaders that disrupt the balance of the body's *doshas* (vital energies) and weaken *Agni* (the digestive fire). This disruption leads to the accumulation of *ama* (toxins), which can manifest as physical illness, mental disturbance, and spiritual disconnection. Ayurveda teaches that parasites are not just a physical affliction but a sign of deeper spiritual and emotional imbalances.

Similarly, in Hinduism and other spiritual traditions, parasites have often been seen as agents of darkness—demonic forces that invade the body, mind, and soul, seeking to corrupt and control. The ancient texts speak of entities that thrive on human suffering, feeding off negative emotions and leading their hosts down paths of self-destruction. These spiritual parasites mirror their biological counterparts, highlighting the interconnectedness of our physical and spiritual worlds.

MEAT PUPPETS: HOW PARASITES CONTROL YOUR BODY, MIND & SPIRIT

ANCIENT WISDOM: THE INDIAN PERSPECTIVE ON PARASITES

The ancient Indians possessed a deep understanding of the ways in which parasites could affect the body, mind, and spirit. Their knowledge was not confined to the physical realm but extended into the metaphysical, recognizing that parasites could be both seen and unseen, physical and spiritual.

In Ayurveda, the science of *Krimi Vidya* (parasitology) provides detailed insights into the causes, symptoms, and treatments of parasitic infestations. The ancient texts describe various types of parasites, categorizing them according to their origins and effects on the body. More importantly, Ayurveda offers a holistic approach to treatment, combining dietary practices, herbal remedies, and detoxification therapies like Panchakarma to cleanse the body of parasites and restore balance.

But Ayurveda does not stop at the physical. It recognizes that parasites are also manifestations of spiritual and emotional disturbances. This understanding is reflected in Hindu practices, where rituals, fasting, and the use of protective herbs are employed to ward off both physical and spiritual parasites. These practices are designed not only to cleanse the body but also to strengthen the mind and spirit, creating a protective shield against negative influences.

THE CONSUMPTION OF MEAT: A GATEWAY TO PARASITIC INFLUENCE

One of the primary ways humans are exposed to parasites is through the consumption of meat. Meat, especially when undercooked or contaminated, is a common source of parasitic infections. But the impact of meat consumption extends beyond the physical. From an Ayurvedic perspective, meat is considered a tamasic food—heavy, inert, and prone to creating toxins in the body. It dulls the mind, weakens the spirit, and opens the door to parasitic influences.

Throughout this book, we will explore how meat consumption compromises human autonomy and spiritual health. We will examine the ways in which parasites, contracted through meat, can manipulate behavior, cloud judgment, and erode spiritual sovereignty. We will also discuss the karmic implications of meat consumption, particularly in the context of Hindu philosophy, where the principle of *ahimsa* (non-violence) is paramount.

As we delve into the connection between parasites and meat consumption, we will uncover the parallels between these physical invaders and the demonic forces described in ancient texts. We will see how parasites, like demons, seek to control and corrupt their hosts, driving them toward behaviors that are harmful to both body and spirit.

RECLAIMING CONTROL OVER OUR HEALTH AND SPIRITUALITY

The subject of this book is clear: the consumption of meat and the resulting exposure to parasites compromise human autonomy and spiritual health. By understanding the nature of parasites, both physical and spiritual, and by adopting practices that protect against their influence, we can reclaim control over our health and spirituality.

This book will guide you through the ancient wisdom of Ayurveda and Hinduism, offering practical tools and insights for cleansing the body, mind, and spirit of parasitic influences. We will explore the role of fasting, a practice that has been largely removed from modern Abrahamic traditions but remains central to Hinduism, as a powerful means of detoxification and spiritual purification. We will also discuss the benefits of adopting a sattvik lifestyle—a life of purity, balance, and spiritual alignment—that minimizes exposure to parasites and fosters spiritual growth.

As we journey together through these chapters, my hope is that you will gain a deeper understanding of the interconnectedness of your physical and spiritual well-being. I encourage you to approach this exploration with an open mind and heart, recognizing that the choices you make in your daily life—what you eat, how you live, and how you connect with the divine—shape not only your physical health but also your spiritual destiny.

Let us embark on this journey of discovery, healing, and empowerment, reclaiming our sovereignty from the parasitic forces that seek to undermine our well-being. Through the wisdom of Ayurveda, Hinduism, and ancient teachings, we can create a life that is in harmony with our highest values, a life that is free, pure, and spiritually sovereign.

With warmth and guidance,

Dr. Sunayana Pandé

PART 2

ANCIENT WISDOM: AYURVEDA AND HINDUISM ON PARASITES

In the vast and intricate tapestry of Ayurveda, the ancient Indian science of life and healing, the study of parasites is known as Krimi Vidya. This knowledge is not limited to the physical understanding of parasites as biological invaders, but it extends into the realms of spiritual and emotional health. Ayurveda views the body, mind, and spirit as deeply interconnected, where disturbances in one aspect inevitably affect the others. In this chapter, we will explore how Ayurveda categorizes and treats parasitic infections, the role of Agni (digestive fire) in maintaining health, and the spiritual implications of parasitic influences.

THE AYURVEDIC PERSPECTIVE ON PARASITES

UNDERSTANDING KRIMI VIDYA: THE SCIENCE OF PARASITES

Ayurveda, with its comprehensive understanding of health and disease, categorizes parasites as *Krimi*. The term *Krimi* broadly refers to any harmful microorganisms, including worms, bacteria, viruses, and other pathogens. These parasites are seen as foreign invaders that disrupt the harmony of the body's *doshas* (Vata,

Pitta, and Kapha) and weaken *Agni*, the vital digestive fire that governs metabolism and immunity.

CLASSIFICATION OF KRIMI (PARASITES)

External and Internal Parasites: Ayurveda classifies *Krimi* into two main categories: external (Bahir Krimi) and internal (Antar Krimi). External parasites include organisms that inhabit the skin and hair, such as lice and scabies, while internal parasites inhabit the gastrointestinal tract, blood, and other internal organs.

Dosha Imbalances: Each type of *Krimi* is associated with specific *dosha* imbalances. For instance, Vata-aggravated parasites cause dryness, constipation, and anxiety; Pitta-aggravated parasites lead to inflammation, fever, and irritability; and Kapha-aggravated parasites result in mucus production, lethargy, and heaviness.

Impact on Agni: The presence of parasites is seen as a sign of weakened *Agni*. When *Agni* is impaired, the body cannot properly digest food, leading to the accumulation of *ama* (toxins). This *ama* creates an environment in which parasites can thrive, further weakening the body and mind.

CAUSES OF PARASITIC INFESTATIONS

Dietary Factors: Ayurveda places significant emphasis on diet as a primary cause of parasitic infestations. The consumption of meat, especially when undercooked or improperly handled, is a major source of parasites. Additionally, foods that are heavy, oily, and difficult to digest—such as processed foods and excessive dairy—can weaken *Agni* and create *ama*, making the body more susceptible to parasites.

Lifestyle Factors: Inadequate sleep, excessive stress, and poor hygiene can also contribute to the development of parasitic infections. A sedentary lifestyle, which slows down metabolism and digestion, further aggravates the risk of parasites taking hold in the body.

Environmental Factors: Exposure to contaminated water, soil, and unclean living conditions are additional factors that increase the risk of parasitic infections. In Ayurveda, the environment is seen as an extension of the self; thus, maintaining a clean and balanced environment is essential for health.

SYMPTOMS OF PARASITIC INFESTATIONS

Physical Symptoms: The symptoms of parasitic infestations vary depending on the type of parasite and the dosha it aggravates. Common physical symptoms include digestive issues (bloating, gas, diarrhea, constipation), skin problems (rashes, itching, lesions), and general signs of toxicity such as fatigue, headaches, and joint pain.

Mental and Emotional Symptoms: Parasitic infestations can also manifest as mental and emotional disturbances. Anxiety, irritability, depression, and even compulsive behaviors can be signs of parasitic influences. Ayurveda recognizes that these symptoms are not just psychological but are often rooted in physical imbalances caused by parasites.

Spiritual Symptoms: On a spiritual level, parasitic infestations can lead to a sense of disconnection from oneself and the divine. Individuals may experience a loss of clarity, purpose, and spiritual direction, feeling as though their vitality and inner light have been dimmed.

AYURVEDIC TREATMENTS FOR PARASITIC INFESTATIONS

Ayurveda offers a holistic approach to treating parasitic infestations, combining dietary modifications, herbal remedies, and detoxification therapies to cleanse the body and restore balance. The goal of treatment is not only to eliminate the parasites but also to strengthen *Agni* and prevent future infestations.

DIETARY PRACTICES

Sattvik Diet: A sattvik diet is light, pure, and easy to digest, helping to restore *Agni* and eliminate *ama*. Foods that are fresh, whole, and naturally grown—such as fruits, vegetables, whole grains, and legumes—are emphasized. These foods nourish the body without creating the conditions in which parasites can thrive.

Avoiding Tamasic Foods: Foods that are heavy, processed, or difficult to digest—classified as tamasic—are to be avoided. This includes meat, processed sugars, refined carbohydrates, and dairy products in excess. These foods weaken *Agni* and contribute to the formation of *ama*, providing a fertile ground for parasites.

Incorporating Digestive Spices: Spices such as ginger, turmeric, cumin, and black pepper are crucial in Ayurvedic treatment for parasites. These spices enhance digestion, boost metabolism, and have natural antimicrobial properties that help to eliminate parasites from the digestive tract.

HERBAL REMEDIES

Vidanga (*Embelia ribes*): Vidanga is a potent herb used in Ayurveda to treat parasitic infections. It has strong anthelmintic properties, meaning it helps to expel worms and other parasites from the body. Vidanga is often used in combination with other herbs to enhance its efficacy.

Neem (*Azadirachta indica*): Neem is another powerful herb with antiparasitic properties. It is used both internally and externally to treat a wide range of parasitic infections. Neem helps to purify the blood, support the immune system, and cleanse the skin and digestive tract.

Haritaki (*Terminalia chebula*): Haritaki is a key ingredient in the Ayurvedic formula Triphala, known for its detoxifying and rejuvenating properties. It helps to regulate digestion, eliminate toxins, and remove parasites from the gastrointestinal tract.

DETOXIFICATION THROUGH PANCHAKARMA

Vamana (Therapeutic Vomiting): Vamana is a cleansing therapy used to expel toxins from the upper digestive tract. It is particularly effective for Kapha-related parasitic infestations, helping to clear mucus, congestion, and other impurities that harbor parasites.

Virechana (Therapeutic Purgation): Virechana involves the use of herbal laxatives to cleanse the liver, intestines, and gallbladder. This therapy is beneficial for Pitta-related conditions, reducing inflammation and eliminating parasites from the lower digestive tract.

Basti (Medicated Enemas): Basti is one of the most powerful Panchakarma therapies, involving the administration of medicated oils or decoctions through the rectum. It is particularly effective for Vata-related disorders, helping to cleanse the colon, remove parasites, and restore balance to the nervous system.

SPIRITUAL AND PHYSICAL INTERCONNECTEDNESS

Ayurveda does not view parasitic infestations solely as physical ailments; they are also seen as manifestations of spiritual and emotional imbalances. This perspective underscores the importance of addressing not just the body but also the mind and spirit in the treatment of parasites.

PARASITES AS MANIFESTATIONS OF IMBALANCE

Spiritual Weakness: In Ayurveda, spiritual weakness or disconnection can make an individual more susceptible to parasitic influences. When one's connection to the divine is weakened, the body's defenses are also compromised, allowing parasites to take hold.

Emotional Disturbances: Negative emotions such as anger, fear, and jealousy are seen as disturbances that weaken the body's natural defenses. These emotions create an environment of toxicity, both internally and externally, making the body more vulnerable to parasites.

STRENGTHENING SPIRITUAL DEFENSES

Mantras and Meditation: Regular meditation and the chanting of mantras are powerful tools for strengthening spiritual defenses. Mantras such as the Mahamrityunjaya Mantra, which invokes Lord Shiva's protection, help to cleanse the mind of negative influences and create a shield against parasitic entities.

Rituals and Offerings: Hindu rituals, such as performing a daily puja or offering prayers to deities, are integral to maintaining spiritual purity. These practices not only protect against physical parasites but also cleanse the mind and spirit of negative energies.

INTEGRATING SPIRITUAL AND PHYSICAL HEALING

Holistic Treatment: Ayurveda's approach to parasitic infestations is holistic, integrating physical treatments with spiritual practices. This combination ensures that the body is cleansed of parasites, the mind is purified of negative thoughts, and the spirit is reconnected with its divine source.

Preventative Care: In addition to treatment, Ayurveda emphasizes the importance of preventative care through lifestyle choices that promote balance and harmony. Regular detoxification, adherence to a sattvik diet, and the practice of yoga and meditation are essential components of this preventative approach.

The Ayurvedic perspective on parasites provides a comprehensive understanding of how these invaders affect not only our physical health but also our mental and spiritual well-being. By recognizing parasites as manifestations of deeper imbalances, Ayurveda offers a holistic approach to treatment that addresses the root causes of infestation.

Through dietary modifications, herbal remedies, and detoxification therapies, Ayurveda provides effective tools for cleansing the body of parasites and restoring balance. However, the true strength of Ayurveda lies in its ability to integrate physical and spiritual healing, ensuring that the mind and spirit are also fortified against parasitic influences.

As we continue this exploration, we will delve deeper into the spiritual dimensions of parasitic influences, examining how they are perceived in Hindu mythology and practices. By understanding these connections, we can develop a more profound appreciation for the wisdom of Ayurveda and its relevance in our modern lives.

In the rich and symbolic world of Hindu mythology, the forces of good and evil are often depicted in a cosmic dance, where gods and demons (Devas and Asuras) represent the eternal struggle between light and darkness, purity and corruption. Parasites, though biological entities, find their echoes in these mythological narratives, embodying the malevolent forces that seek to disrupt the harmony of life and spirituality. In this chapter, we will explore the references to parasitic influences in Hindu mythology, draw parallels between these ancient stories and the physical reality of parasitic infections, and delve into the traditional Hindu practices designed to protect against and combat these insidious forces.

PARASITES IN HINDU MYTHOLOGY AND PRACTICES

MYTHOLOGICAL REFERENCES: THE PARASITIC INFLUENCE IN HINDU LORE

Hindu mythology is filled with tales of Asuras, Rakshasas, and other malevolent beings who embody the darker aspects of existence. These entities often symbolize the internal and external forces that seek to undermine dharma (righteousness) and lead individuals away from the path of spiritual growth. Just as parasites invade the body, these demonic forces invade the mind and spirit, corrupting thoughts, behaviors, and spiritual inclinations.

ASURAS AND PARASITES: THE FORCES OF CORRUPTION

Asuras in Hindu Mythology: Asuras are often depicted as powerful beings with immense strength and intelligence, but their motivations are driven by greed, pride, and a desire to dominate. They represent the forces of *adharma* (unrighteousness) that oppose the gods and seek to disrupt the balance of the universe.

Parasitic Parallels: The behavior of Asuras can be compared to that of parasites, which invade their hosts, drain their vitality, and lead them toward destruction. Just as Asuras are obsessed with power and control, parasites manipulate their hosts, often leading to physical and mental deterioration.

The Tale of Vritra: In one of the Puranic stories, Vritra, a powerful Asura, takes control of the waters of the world, causing drought and suffering. Indra, the king of the gods, ultimately defeats Vritra, symbolizing the triumph of righteousness over corruption. This story can be seen as an allegory for how parasitic influences can control vital resources (like the body's energy) and how they must be overcome to restore balance.

RAKSHASAS AND SPIRITUAL PARASITISM

Rakshasas in Hindu Mythology: Rakshasas are another class of malevolent beings often portrayed as flesh-eating demons with insatiable appetites for destruction. They are typically associated with darkness, chaos, and the disruption of dharma. Some Rakshasas, like Ravana in the Ramayana, possess great intellect and power but use these gifts for destructive purposes.

Parasitic Behavior: Rakshasas, like parasites, feed off the life force of others, consuming not just their physical resources but also their mental and spiritual energies. They represent the forces of greed, lust, and gluttony—traits that are often exacerbated by parasitic infestations in the physical world.

The Story of Surpanakha: In the Ramayana, Surpanakha, the sister of Ravana, symbolizes unchecked desire and the destructive consequences of parasitic behavior. Her actions lead to her downfall, as well as the eventual destruction of her brother's empire. This narrative highlights the dangers of succumbing to parasitic influences, whether they are external demons or internal cravings driven by parasitic entities.

NAGAS AND THE DUAL NATURE OF SERPENTS

Nagas in Hindu Mythology: Nagas are serpentine beings with a dual nature; they can be protectors and sources of wisdom, but they can also be destructive forces. In some myths, Nagas are associated with the underworld and are believed to guard treasures, both material and spiritual.

Serpents as Symbols of Parasites: The serpent, a symbol often associated with both wisdom and danger, can be seen as a metaphor for parasites. Just as some serpents are venomous, some parasites carry toxins that can corrupt the body and mind. The duality of the serpent—both revered and feared—mirrors the duality of parasites, which can be subtle yet deadly.

The Churning of the Ocean (Samudra Manthan): In the myth of Samudra Manthan, the serpent Vasuki is used as a rope in the cosmic churning of the ocean, which produces both nectar (Amrita) and poison (Halahala). This story symbolizes the dual nature of life, where both positive and negative forces coexist. Parasites, like the poison from the churning, represent the negative forces that must be managed and neutralized to attain balance and purity.

CONNECTING MYTHOLOGICAL REFERENCES TO PHYSICAL REALITY

The ancient stories of Asuras, Rakshasas, and Nagas are more than just mythological tales; they offer profound insights into the nature of human existence and the challenges we face in maintaining physical, mental, and spiritual health. By examining these myths through the lens of parasitic influences, we can better understand the ways in which parasites operate and how they affect our lives.

PARALLELS BETWEEN MYTH AND PARASITIC INFECTIONS

Invasion and Control: Just as Asuras and Rakshasas invade the realms of gods and humans, parasites invade the human body, seeking to control its resources for their benefit. The struggle between gods and demons mirrors the internal struggle we face when dealing with parasitic infections—whether those parasites are physical organisms or negative thoughts and behaviors.

Manipulation of Behavior: Many parasites are known to manipulate the behavior of their hosts to ensure their survival and propagation. This can be likened to the influence of demonic forces in mythology, which manipulate individuals to act against their better judgment, leading to their downfall.

The Battle for Purity: In Hindu mythology, the gods often engage in battles to protect dharma and restore balance. Similarly, the body engages in a constant battle to maintain purity and health, defending against the invasion of parasites and other harmful influences.

SPIRITUAL CONSEQUENCES OF PARASITIC INFLUENCES

Loss of Autonomy: Just as demonic forces in mythology seek to enslave or dominate, parasites can rob individuals of their autonomy by influencing their thoughts, desires, and actions. This loss of control can lead to a sense of spiritual disconnection and despair.

Erosion of Dharma: Parasites, much like the Asuras, erode dharma by creating chaos within the body and mind. They disrupt the natural balance, leading to physical illness, mental confusion, and spiritual degradation. Over time, this erosion can weaken an individual's resolve to follow the path of righteousness and self-discipline.

The Need for Divine Intervention: In many myths, divine intervention is required to defeat the Asuras and restore order. Similarly, overcoming parasitic influences often requires a combination of physical, mental, and spiritual practices—drawing on the divine within us to cleanse and protect ourselves from harm.

HINDU PRACTICES FOR PROTECTION

Hinduism offers a wealth of practices designed to protect against both physical and spiritual parasitic influences. These practices are rooted in a deep understanding of the interconnectedness of body, mind, and spirit, and they provide a holistic approach to maintaining health and spiritual sovereignty.

FASTING (UPAVASA)

The Purifying Power of Fasting: Fasting is one of the most powerful practices in Hinduism for cleansing the body and spirit. Regular fasting, whether on specific holy days or as part of a spiritual discipline, helps to detoxify the body, expel parasites, and purify the mind.

Fasting and Parasite Removal: From an Ayurvedic perspective, fasting helps to strengthen *Agni* and burn off *ama*, creating an environment in which parasites cannot survive. By abstaining from food, the body is given the opportunity to reset and rejuvenate, eliminating toxins and restoring balance.

Fasting as a Spiritual Practice: Beyond its physical benefits, fasting is also a profound spiritual practice that fosters self-discipline, humility, and devotion. It is a way of offering one's physical needs to the divine, seeking spiritual clarity and protection from harmful influences.

THE USE OF PROTECTIVE HERBS

Neem (*Azadirachta indica*): Neem, known as the "village pharmacy," is a sacred plant in Hinduism with powerful antiparasitic properties. It is used in various forms—leaves, oil, and extracts—to cleanse the body, purify the blood, and protect against infections. In Hindu rituals, neem is often used to purify the environment and protect against evil spirits.

Tulsi (Holy Basil): Tulsi, revered as a manifestation of the goddess Lakshmi, is another powerful herb used for protection. It has strong antimicrobial properties and is used to boost immunity, clear toxins, and protect the home from negative energies. Tulsi leaves are often offered in pujas and are considered essential in maintaining spiritual purity.

Vidanga (*Embelia ribes*): Vidanga is specifically used in Ayurveda to expel intestinal worms and other parasites. It is often included in formulas for detoxification and cleansing, helping to restore balance to the digestive system and eliminate harmful organisms.

THE ROLE OF AGNI (FIRE) IN HINDU RITUALS

Agni as a Purifier: In Hinduism, fire is a symbol of transformation and purification. Agni, the fire god, is invoked in rituals to purify offerings, cleanse spaces, and protect against evil forces. The practice of *Agnihotra*—offering ghee and grains into the sacred fire—helps to neutralize negative energies and parasites, both physical and spiritual.

Agni and Digestive Fire: Just as Agni purifies in rituals, the digestive fire (also called Agni) is responsible for purifying the body. A strong digestive fire is essential for breaking down food, assimilating nutrients, and burning off toxins and parasites. Maintaining Agni through diet, herbs, and fasting is central to both physical and spiritual health.

Fire Rituals (Yajnas): Yajnas, or fire sacrifices, are integral to Hindu worship. These rituals involve offering various substances into the sacred fire while chanting mantras. The fire is believed to carry the offerings to the gods, purifying the environment and the participants. Yajnas are performed to seek protection, health, and spiritual growth, creating a barrier against parasitic and demonic influences.

Parasites, both physical and spiritual, have been recognized throughout Hindu mythology and practices as forces that seek to disrupt the natural order and lead individuals away from the path of dharma. By understanding these influences and their manifestations, we can better equip ourselves to combat them.

Hindu practices offer a comprehensive approach to protecting against parasitic influences, emphasizing the importance of purification, fasting, and the use of protective herbs. These practices are not just about maintaining physical health; they are also about safeguarding the mind and spirit, ensuring that we remain aligned with our highest selves and the divine.

As we move forward in this book, we will continue to explore how these ancient practices can be applied in modern life, offering practical tools for reclaiming control over our health and spiritual well-being. By drawing on the wisdom of Hindu mythology and practices, we can strengthen our defenses against the parasitic forces that seek to undermine our autonomy and spiritual sovereignty.

PART 3

THE DEMONIC PARALLELS: PARASITES ACROSS CULTURES

Cats have long held a unique place in human history, mythology, and spirituality. Revered in some cultures and feared in others, these enigmatic creatures have been associated with both protective and malevolent forces. In Hinduism, cats are seen as both spiritual entities and symbols of independence, intuition, and mystery. However, their role in human health and spirituality becomes even more complex when we consider their relationship with Toxoplasma gondii—a parasitic organism that thrives in the bodies of cats and can have profound effects on human behavior and health. This chapter explores the multifaceted role of cats in Hindu culture, their significance in Ayurveda, and the scientific understanding of their role as hosts of Toxoplasma gondii.

CATS IN HINDUISM, AYURVEDA, AND PARASITOLOGY

CATS AS SPIRITUAL ENTITIES IN HINDUISM

In Hindu culture, animals are often viewed as manifestations of the divine, and each species carries its own symbolic meaning. Cats, with their graceful movements and keen senses, are no exception. They are seen as symbols of mystery, independence, and spiritual insight, often associated with the goddess Shashthi, the protector of children and fertility.

THE ROLE OF CATS IN HINDU MYTHOLOGY

Goddess Shashthi: In Hindu mythology, the goddess Shashthi is often depicted riding a cat. She is revered as the protector of children and the goddess of fertility and childbirth. The cat, as her vahana (vehicle), symbolizes the protective and nurturing aspects of the goddess. Shashthi is invoked by mothers to ensure the safety and well-being of their children, and her association with the cat highlights the animal's role as a guardian.

Cats and Intuition: Cats are also seen as symbols of intuition and mysticism. Their nocturnal habits and ability to see in the dark are often associated with the ability to perceive hidden truths and navigate the spiritual realms. In this sense, cats are considered to be in tune with the unseen world, making them powerful symbols of spiritual awareness.

The Duality of Cats: Despite their revered status, cats are also seen as creatures of duality in Hinduism. They embody both the nurturing and protective aspects of the divine, as well as the mysterious and sometimes unsettling qualities associated with the unknown. This duality is reflected in their association with both positive and negative forces in various cultural traditions.

CATS IN HINDU RITUALS AND DAILY LIFE

Cats as Household Protectors: In Hindu households, cats are often seen as protectors of the home, keeping away pests and negative energies. Their presence is believed to create a protective barrier that wards off evil spirits and malevolent influences. This belief is rooted in the idea that cats have a natural ability to sense and repel negative energies.

Rituals Involving Cats: Cats are occasionally involved in Hindu rituals, particularly those related to fertility and protection. For example, offerings might be made to a cat or the goddess Shashthi to invoke blessings for children or to ensure the safety of the home. In some regions, it is considered auspicious to care for stray cats as a way of gaining favor with the goddess.

Superstitions and Beliefs: While cats are generally seen as positive figures, certain superstitions also surround them. For example, it is believed that a cat crossing one's path can be a sign of impending danger or misfortune, though this belief varies by region. These superstitions underscore the complex relationship between humans and cats, blending reverence with caution.

THE AYURVEDIC VIEW ON CATS

In Ayurveda, the holistic system of health and wellness that originated in ancient India, animals play a significant role in human health, both as companions and as potential sources of imbalance. The Ayurvedic view of cats, particularly in relation to health and hygiene, is shaped by their role as carriers of certain parasites, most notably *Toxoplasma gondii*.

THE IMPORTANCE OF CLEANLINESS AND HYGIENE

Ayurvedic Principles of Hygiene: Ayurveda places great emphasis on cleanliness (Shaucha) as a fundamental principle of health. This extends to the cleanliness of the home and surroundings, which is believed to directly impact one's physical and mental well-being. Animals, including cats, are seen as part of this environment, and their cleanliness is considered essential to maintaining balance and health.

Cats and Hygiene Practices: While cats are known for their grooming habits, their role as potential carriers of parasites like *Toxoplasma gondii* requires careful consideration. In Ayurvedic practices, maintaining a clean environment where animals are present is crucial to preventing the spread of infections. This includes regular cleaning of areas where cats reside, ensuring they are well cared for, and maintaining personal hygiene after handling them.

The Role of Diet and Environment: Ayurveda also recognizes the impact of diet and environment on the health of both humans and animals. A sattvik diet, which is pure and balanced, is recommended for those who keep pets, as it helps to maintain the health of both the owner and the animal. Similarly, the environment should be kept clean and free from impurities, which can harbor parasites and other pathogens.

THE AYURVEDIC PERSPECTIVE ON ANIMAL INTERACTIONS

Balance and Dosha Interactions: In Ayurveda, interactions with animals are seen through the lens of doshas (Vata, Pitta, and Kapha). Cats, with their agile and independent nature, are often associated with Vata energy. Excessive interaction with cats, especially for those with a Vata imbalance, may lead to increased anxiety, restlessness, and nervousness. Therefore, Ayurveda recommends moderation and balance in all interactions with animals.

Herbal Remedies for Pet Owners: Ayurveda suggests certain herbal remedies and practices for those who live with animals to maintain balance and prevent health issues. For example, burning dried neem leaves or using neem oil in the home can help purify the air and reduce the risk of parasitic infections. Similarly, using turmeric, a natural antiseptic, in cleaning practices can further protect against potential pathogens.

TOXOPLASMA GONDII AND THE SPIRITUAL CONNECTION

One of the most fascinating and concerning aspects of the relationship between cats and human health is their role as the definitive hosts of *Toxoplasma gondii*, a parasitic protozoan that can have profound effects on human behavior and spirituality. This section explores the biological and spiritual implications of this parasite, drawing connections between ancient beliefs and modern science.

UNDERSTANDING TOXOPLASMA GONDII

Lifecycle and Transmission: *Toxoplasma gondii* has a complex lifecycle that requires felines, particularly domestic cats, as definitive hosts. The parasite reproduces sexually within the intestines of cats and is then shed in their feces as oocysts. These oocysts can survive in the environment for long periods, potentially infecting humans through contaminated soil, water, or undercooked meat.

Behavioral Manipulation: Scientific studies have shown that *T. gondii* can manipulate the behavior of its hosts to increase its chances of transmission. In rodents, for example, the parasite reduces the natural fear of predators, making them more likely to be caught by cats. In humans, *T. gondii* has been linked to various behavioral changes, including increased risk-taking, impulsivity, and, in some cases, symptoms similar to those seen in schizophrenia.

Health Implications: While many people infected with *T. gondii* may remain asymptomatic, the parasite can cause serious health issues in certain individuals, particularly those with weakened immune systems. These can include neurological disorders, vision problems, and in severe cases, life-threatening infections.

TOXOPLASMA GONDII AS A MODERN PARALLEL TO ANCIENT BELIEFS

Demonic Possession and Behavioral Changes: The behavioral manipulation caused by *T. gondii* can be seen as a modern parallel to ancient beliefs about demonic possession. In many cultures, sudden changes in behavior, particularly those involving risk-taking or irrational fears, were attributed to malevolent spiritual forces. The ability of *T. gondii* to influence human behavior echoes these ancient fears, suggesting a link between parasitic infection and what might be perceived as spiritual or demonic influence.

The Spiritual Consequences of Infection: From a spiritual perspective, the influence of *T. gondii* can be seen as a form of possession or hijacking of the soul. The parasite's ability to alter behavior, reduce fear, and increase attraction to dangerous or harmful situations can lead to a loss of spiritual clarity and autonomy. In this sense, infection by *T. gondii* represents not just a physical health risk but a threat to one's spiritual well-being and connection to the divine.

The Role of Cats as Spiritual Intermediaries: Given their role as definitive hosts for *T. gondii*, cats occupy a unique position in the intersection of health, spirituality, and mythology. In ancient cultures, including those of Egypt and Hinduism, cats were often seen as intermediaries between the human and spiritual realms. The discovery of *T. gondii* reinforces this connection, suggesting that cats may indeed serve as conduits for both physical and spiritual influences.

THE BROADER IMPLICATIONS OF TOXOPLASMA GONDII

Impact on Society: The widespread presence of *T. gondii* has significant implications for society as a whole. Studies suggest that a large portion of the global population is infected with the parasite, often unknowingly. This raises questions about the subtle ways in which parasites may be influencing behavior on a larger scale, potentially affecting decision-making, social dynamics, and even cultural norms.

Ethical Considerations: The relationship between humans, cats, and *T. gondii* also prompts ethical considerations. How should we balance our reverence for cats as spiritual entities with the need to protect human health? What responsibilities do pet owners have in preventing the spread of this parasite? These questions highlight the complex interplay between tradition, science, and ethics in our interactions with the natural world.

CATS, PARASITES, AND THE SPIRITUAL DIMENSION

The relationship between cats, parasites, and human spirituality is a deeply complex and multifaceted one. Cats, revered in Hinduism and other ancient cultures as spiritual beings, also serve as hosts for *Toxoplasma gondii*, a parasite that can influence human behavior in ways that eerily echo the concept of demonic possession.

THE PROTECTIVE ROLE OF CATS

Guardians of the Home: Despite the potential risks associated with *T. gondii*, cats continue to be seen as protectors of the home in Hindu culture. Their presence is believed to ward off negative energies and protect against evil spirits. This duality—where cats are both potential carriers of a harmful parasite and revered as spiritual guardians—reflects the broader theme of balance in Hinduism, where light and dark, positive and negative, coexist and must be managed with wisdom and care.

Spiritual Intermediaries: Cats' role as intermediaries between the physical and spiritual realms suggests that they may help facilitate a deeper connection with the divine. However, this role also requires careful management of the physical risks they pose, particularly in relation to parasites like *T. gondii*.

ADDRESSING THE SPIRITUAL AND PHYSICAL RISKS

Ayurvedic Practices for Protection: Ayurveda offers practical solutions for addressing the risks associated with cats and *T. gondii*. These include maintaining cleanliness, using herbal remedies like neem and turmeric, and practicing regular detoxification. These practices help to minimize the physical risks while honoring the spiritual role of cats in the household.

Balancing Reverence with Responsibility: Hindus are encouraged to balance their reverence for cats with the responsibility of protecting themselves and their families from potential health risks. This involves not only maintaining hygiene but also fostering a sattvik lifestyle that supports overall health and spiritual clarity.

INTEGRATING ANCIENT WISDOM WITH MODERN UNDERSTANDING

The Evolution of Beliefs: The discovery of *T. gondii* offers a fascinating lens through which to reinterpret ancient beliefs about cats and their role in human life. By integrating this modern understanding with traditional Hindu practices, we can develop a more holistic approach to health and spirituality.

Continued Reverence: Even as we acknowledge the risks associated with *T. gondii*, it is important to maintain our reverence for cats as spiritual beings. Their presence in our lives serves as a reminder of the deep interconnectedness between the physical and spiritual worlds, and the need to approach both with respect, care, and wisdom.

Cats have long been seen as mysterious and powerful creatures in Hindu culture, embodying both protective and potentially dangerous qualities. Their role as hosts for *Toxoplasma gondii* adds a new dimension to our understanding of their influence on human health and spirituality. By examining the connections between cats, parasites, and human behavior through the lenses of Ayurveda, Hinduism, and modern science, we can develop a more nuanced appreciation for these enigmatic animals.

As we continue to explore the parasitic influences on human life, we must balance our reverence for cats as spiritual entities with the responsibility of protecting ourselves from the risks they may pose. By integrating ancient wisdom with modern understanding, we can navigate this complex relationship in a way that honors both our health and our spiritual traditions.

Throughout history, parasites have been understood not only as biological entities but also as symbols of spiritual corruption and demonic influence. In various cultures and religious traditions, the impact of parasites on the human body has often been linked to the presence of malevolent forces seeking to undermine physical, mental, and spiritual well-being. This chapter explores the biblical perspectives on parasites, their portrayal as demonic influences, and how these views align with or differ from cultural beliefs around the world. We will also delve into the significant yet often overlooked removal of fasting from modern biblical practices and its implications for spiritual and physical health.

THE BIBLICAL AND CULTURAL VIEWS OF PARASITES

BIBLICAL PERSPECTIVES ON PARASITES AS DEMONIC INFLUENCES

The Bible, particularly in its older texts, frequently associates disease, filth, and corruption with demonic forces. Parasites, as agents of disease, are often seen through a similar lens—as physical manifestations of spiritual decay. These ancient views offer profound insights into how parasites were perceived in a religious context and the spiritual significance attributed to their presence.

BEELZEBUB: THE LORD OF THE FLIES

Beelzebub in the Bible: One of the most prominent biblical figures associated with filth, disease, and demonic influence is Beelzebub, whose name means "Lord of the Flies" in Hebrew. Beelzebub is often depicted as a powerful demon or prince of demons in the New Testament, particularly in the Gospel of Matthew. His association with flies—a creature known for spreading disease—highlights the biblical view of parasites and pests as carriers of demonic energy.

Lord of Filth and Disease: Beelzebub's title, "Lord of the Flies," is a direct reference to his dominion over filth and decay, environments where parasites thrive. In ancient times, flies were a common carrier of diseases and parasites, particularly in areas with poor sanitation. The biblical portrayal of Beelzebub as a demonic figure ruling over such conditions underscores the belief that parasites and their carriers are not merely physical nuisances but embodiments of spiritual corruption.

Cultural Parallels: The association of flies and other pests with demonic influence is not unique to the Bible. Similar beliefs are found in various cultures, where flies and other insects are seen as symbols of decay, death, and the presence of evil spirits. In Egyptian mythology, for example, flies were considered to be the minions of Set, the god of chaos and destruction.

THE THREE WORMS: DAOIST BELIEFS AND THEIR CONNECTIONS

Daoist Concept of the Three Worms: In Daoist beliefs, the "Three Worms" (San Shi or Shi) are demonic creatures that reside within the human body, feeding off the host's vital energy and causing illness, decay, and ultimately death. These worms are said to report the sins of their host to the gods, hastening their demise. The concept of the Three Worms reflects an understanding of parasites as both physical and spiritual entities that undermine health and morality.

Parasitic Parallels: The Daoist concept of the Three Worms closely parallels the biblical view of parasites as agents of spiritual corruption. Both traditions emphasize the destructive influence of these entities on the body and soul, suggesting that physical illness and moral decay are interconnected.

Cultural Transmission: The idea that parasites and worms could be manifestations of spiritual or demonic forces likely spread through cultural exchanges along trade routes such as the Silk Road. These beliefs were incorporated into various religious traditions, leading to a shared understanding of parasites as symbols of moral and physical decay.

THE SERPENT AND THE FALL: SYMBOLISM OF PARASITES IN GENESIS

The Serpent in the Garden of Eden: The serpent in the Garden of Eden, who tempts Eve to eat the forbidden fruit, is one of the most iconic symbols of sin and demonic influence in the Bible. While the serpent itself is not a parasite, its role as a deceiver and corrupter mirrors the behavior of parasites, which invade the body and manipulate their hosts for their own gain.

Symbolic Interpretation: In a symbolic sense, the serpent can be seen as a metaphor for parasitic influences—entities that introduce corruption into the human soul, leading to spiritual death. Just as the serpent leads Adam and Eve away from their pure state of being, parasites lead the body away from health and balance, causing both physical and spiritual harm.

The Curse of the Serpent: After the fall, God curses the serpent to crawl on its belly and eat dust for the rest of its days. This curse can be interpreted as a reflection of the parasitic nature of evil—forever bound to the earth, feeding off the remnants of life, and spreading corruption wherever it goes.

THE REMOVAL OF FASTING FROM THE BIBLE: SPIRITUAL AND PHYSICAL CONSEQUENCES

Fasting has long been a crucial practice in many religious traditions, including Christianity, as a means of purifying the body and soul. However, in modern times, the emphasis on fasting has diminished, particularly in Western Christianity. This shift has significant implications for both spiritual and physical health, especially in the context of protecting against parasitic influences.

FASTING IN BIBLICAL TRADITION

Fasting as a Spiritual Discipline: In the Bible, fasting is frequently mentioned as a way to seek divine guidance, repent for sins, and purify oneself spiritually. Jesus himself fasted for 40 days and nights in the wilderness, resisting the temptations of Satan and emerging spiritually strengthened. This practice is seen as a means of drawing closer to God by denying the physical body and focusing on the spiritual.

Fasting and Protection: Fasting is not just about spiritual discipline; it is also seen as a way to protect oneself from evil influences. By fasting, believers cleanse their bodies of impurities, making themselves less susceptible to demonic attacks or spiritual corruption. This idea is echoed in the practices of many cultures, where fasting is used to ward off illness, evil spirits, and negative energies.

THE DIMINISHED ROLE OF FASTING IN MODERN CHRISTIANITY

Changes in Biblical Texts: Over time, the emphasis on fasting has been significantly reduced in many modern Christian denominations. Some versions of the Bible, particularly the New International Version (NIV) and the English Standard Version (ESV), have even removed or altered references to fasting. For example, in Matthew 17:21, which originally stated that certain demons could only be cast out through prayer and fasting, modern translations often omit the fasting component.

Spiritual Vulnerability: The removal of fasting from modern Christian practices has left many believers spiritually vulnerable. Without this critical discipline, the body and soul are more susceptible to parasitic influences—both physical parasites that thrive on impurities and spiritual parasites that corrupt the mind and spirit. This shift away from fasting represents a loss of an essential tool for maintaining spiritual sovereignty and protection.

THE SONS OF ABRAHAM AND PARASITIC VULNERABILITY

A Historical Perspective: The sons of Abraham—Jews, Christians, and Muslims—have historically been guided by divine laws designed to protect them physically and spiritually. However, as these traditions have evolved, some of these protective practices, such as fasting, have been diminished or forgotten. This erosion of spiritual discipline has left the followers of these traditions more vulnerable to parasitic influences.

Parasitic Influence and Spiritual Decline: The decline of fasting and other purificatory practices in the Abrahamic religions may be linked to an increase in physical and spiritual ailments among their followers. Without regular fasting, the body accumulates toxins and becomes a more hospitable environment for parasites, both biological and spiritual. This vulnerability can lead to a decline in spiritual clarity, moral discipline, and overall health.

The Enduring Practice of Fasting in Hinduism: In contrast, fasting remains a central practice in Hinduism, where it is used not only for spiritual purification but also as a means of maintaining physical health and preventing parasitic infestations. The continued emphasis on fasting in Hindu culture has helped its followers maintain spiritual sovereignty and minimize exposure to parasitic influences.

CULTURAL BELIEFS ABOUT PARASITES AND THEIR SPIRITUAL SIGNIFICANCE

Beyond the Abrahamic religions, many cultures around the world have their own beliefs about parasites and their spiritual significance. These beliefs often reflect a deep understanding of the interconnectedness of physical and spiritual health, and they offer valuable insights into how different societies have addressed the challenge of parasitic influences.

PARASITES AS SYMBOLS OF CORRUPTION

African Traditions: In many African cultures, parasites are seen as symbols of moral and spiritual corruption. Traditional healers, known as sangomas or shamans, often treat parasitic infections as manifestations of spiritual imbalance. Rituals and herbal treatments are used not only to expel the parasites but also to restore the patient's spiritual harmony.

Indigenous Beliefs in the Americas: Among indigenous peoples in the Americas, parasites are often associated with negative spiritual forces or curses. Shamans may use fasting, herbal remedies, and spiritual cleansing rituals to treat parasitic infections, emphasizing the need to purify both the body and the spirit. In some traditions, certain parasites are believed to be sent by malevolent spirits to punish or test individuals.

Asian Perspectives: In East Asian cultures, particularly in traditional Chinese medicine, parasites are seen as a result of imbalances in the body's energy (Qi). These imbalances are often linked to moral or spiritual issues, and treatment involves restoring harmony to the body's internal environment. The use of fasting, detoxification, and herbal medicine is common in these traditions, reflecting a holistic approach to health.

THE ROLE OF RITUALS AND PROTECTIVE PRACTICES

Rituals for Purification: Across cultures, rituals play a key role in protecting against parasitic influences. These rituals often involve purification through fasting, prayer, and the use of sacred herbs or substances. In many cases, these practices are intended to cleanse not only the body but also the soul, driving out negative energies and restoring spiritual balance.

Protective Symbols and Amulets: In addition to rituals, many cultures use protective symbols and amulets to ward off parasites and evil spirits. These items are often blessed or consecrated by religious leaders and are believed to create a barrier against harmful influences. In some traditions, certain animals, such as cats or snakes, are also revered as protectors against parasites and spiritual corruption.

THE INTEGRATION OF MODERN SCIENCE AND TRADITIONAL BELIEFS

Scientific Understanding of Parasites: Modern science has provided a deeper understanding of the biology of parasites and their impact on human health. However, this knowledge does not diminish the importance of traditional beliefs and practices. Instead, it offers an opportunity to integrate scientific insights with spiritual and cultural wisdom, creating a more comprehensive approach to health and well-being.

Holistic Approaches to Health: By combining modern medical treatments with traditional practices such as fasting, herbal medicine, and spiritual cleansing, individuals can protect themselves against both the physical and spiritual aspects of parasitic infections. This holistic approach recognizes that true health encompasses the body, mind, and spirit, and that all three must be nurtured and protected.

THE SATTVIK LIFESTYLE: MINIMIZING EXPOSURE TO PARASITES

In contrast to the diminished emphasis on fasting in many Abrahamic traditions, Hinduism has preserved the practice of fasting as a central tenet of its spiritual discipline. This commitment to regular purification and a sattvik lifestyle has helped Hindus maintain both physical and spiritual health, minimizing their exposure to parasitic influences.

THE SATTVIK DIET

Purity and Simplicity: The sattvik diet, which emphasizes purity, simplicity, and balance, is designed to promote health and spiritual clarity. By avoiding tamasic foods—those that are heavy, processed, and difficult to digest—Hindus minimize the risk of creating an environment in which parasites can thrive. Instead, they focus on fresh fruits, vegetables, whole grains, and dairy products that support digestion and nourish the body without contributing to the accumulation of toxins.

Herbs and Spices: The use of herbs and spices such as turmeric, ginger, and neem in the sattvik diet also plays a crucial role in preventing parasitic infections. These natural ingredients have powerful antimicrobial and antiparasitic properties, helping to cleanse the body and support the immune system.

FASTING AS A REGULAR PRACTICE

Monthly and Weekly Fasts: Fasting is deeply ingrained in Hindu culture, with many Hindus observing regular fasts on specific days of the week or month, such as Ekadashi or Purnima. These fasts serve not only as spiritual disciplines but also as powerful tools for detoxification and health maintenance. By giving the digestive system a rest and allowing the body to cleanse itself, fasting helps to eliminate toxins and parasites, promoting overall well-being.

Spiritual Benefits of Fasting: Beyond its physical benefits, fasting is also seen as a way to strengthen one's connection with the divine. By denying the physical body and focusing on spiritual practices, individuals can purify their minds, increase their self-discipline, and enhance their spiritual awareness. This holistic approach to fasting recognizes the interconnectedness of body, mind, and spirit, ensuring that all aspects of health are addressed.

THE ROLE OF RITUALS AND SPIRITUAL PRACTICES

Daily Rituals for Protection: In addition to fasting and diet, Hinduism emphasizes the importance of daily rituals for maintaining spiritual and physical health. These rituals often involve the use of sacred herbs, mantras, and offerings to deities, creating a protective environment that wards off negative influences and parasites. For example, the burning of camphor or incense during puja is believed to purify the air and repel harmful entities.

Spiritual Sovereignty: By maintaining a sattvik lifestyle and regularly practicing fasting, Hindus are able to maintain their spiritual sovereignty and resist the influence of parasitic forces. This commitment to purity and discipline ensures that both the body and spirit remain strong and resilient, capable of withstanding the challenges of the physical and spiritual worlds.

The relationship between parasites and spiritual health is a theme that resonates across cultures and religious traditions. In the Bible and other cultural beliefs, parasites are often seen as symbols of moral and physical corruption, linked to demonic influences and spiritual decay. The removal of fasting from modern Christian practices has left many believers vulnerable to these influences, while the continued emphasis on fasting and purity in Hinduism has helped to protect its followers from both physical and spiritual harm.

As we continue to explore the impact of parasites on human health and spirituality, it is essential to recognize the importance of maintaining practices that cleanse and purify the body and soul. By integrating traditional beliefs with modern scientific understanding, we can develop a more holistic approach to health—one that addresses the physical, mental, and spiritual aspects of our being. In doing so, we can protect ourselves from the parasitic forces that seek to undermine our health and spiritual sovereignty, ensuring that we remain strong, balanced, and connected to the divine.

PART 4

THE PARASITIC INFLUENCE ON BEHAVIOR AND SPIRITUAL HEALTH

The relationship between parasites and their hosts is one of the most fascinating and disturbing aspects of biology. Parasites have evolved highly specialized mechanisms to manipulate the behavior of their hosts, ensuring their own survival and propagation. These manipulations can range from subtle changes in mood and appetite to drastic alterations in risk-taking behavior and sexual attraction. In this chapter, we will explore the scientific evidence linking parasites to changes in human behavior, examine the broader implications of these findings, and discuss these behaviors through a spiritual lens, drawing parallels to the influence of demonic forces.

HOW PARASITES MANIPULATE HUMAN BEHAVIOR

TOXOPLASMA GONDII AND BEHAVIORAL CHANGES

One of the most well-documented examples of a parasite manipulating its host's behavior is *Toxoplasma gondii*, a protozoan parasite that primarily infects cats but can also infect humans. The behavioral changes induced by *T. gondii* provide a striking example of how parasites can influence not only physical health but also mental and emotional well-being.

THE LIFECYCLE OF TOXOPLASMA GONDII

Transmission and Infection: *Toxoplasma gondii* has a complex lifecycle that involves both felines and a variety of intermediate hosts, including rodents, birds, and humans. The parasite reproduces sexually within the intestines of cats, and its oocysts are shed in their feces. These oocysts can contaminate soil, water, and food, leading to infection in other animals and humans.

Behavioral Manipulation in Rodents: Infected rodents exhibit a range of behavioral changes that increase their likelihood of being preyed upon by cats, thereby completing the parasite's lifecycle. One of the most notable changes is the loss of fear of cat odor, which normally deters rodents from entering areas frequented by cats. Instead, infected rodents may be attracted to these areas, making them easy targets for predation.

BEHAVIORAL CHANGES IN HUMANS

Increased Risk-Taking: In humans, *T. gondii* infection has been associated with a variety of behavioral changes, including increased risk-taking behavior. Studies have shown that infected individuals are more likely to engage in risky activities, such as reckless driving or dangerous sports. This increased propensity for risk-taking may be a result of the parasite's influence on the brain's dopamine system, which plays a key role in reward and risk assessment.

Attraction to Danger: *T. gondii* infection has also been linked to an increased attraction to danger and novelty. Infected individuals may be more likely to seek out thrilling or dangerous experiences, which could increase their chances of harm. This behavior mirrors the effects seen in rodents and suggests that the parasite may manipulate the brain's reward circuits to encourage behaviors that facilitate its transmission.

Changes in Personality: Some studies have suggested that *T. gondii* infection can lead to subtle changes in personality, such as increased impulsivity, aggression, and even symptoms of mental disorders like schizophrenia. These changes may be related to the parasite's impact on the brain's neurotransmitter systems, including dopamine and serotonin.

THE SPIRITUAL INTERPRETATION OF TOXOPLASMA GONDII'S INFLUENCE

Parallels to Demonic Possession: The behavioral changes induced by *T. gondii* can be viewed through a spiritual lens as a form of demonic possession. Just as demonic forces are believed to manipulate individuals to act against their better judgment, *T.*

gondii manipulates its host's behavior in ways that serve the parasite's interests rather than the host's well-being. This manipulation of behavior can lead to a loss of autonomy, making individuals more susceptible to negative influences.

The Erosion of Free Will: From a spiritual perspective, the influence of *T. gondii* represents a subtle erosion of free will. The parasite's ability to alter behavior without the host's conscious awareness mirrors the way negative spiritual influences can lead individuals away from their true path. This erosion of free will can have profound consequences for both physical and spiritual health, leading to a sense of disconnection and loss of purpose.

Spiritual Vulnerability: The presence of *T. gondii* in the body may create a state of spiritual vulnerability, where the individual is more susceptible to other negative influences, both physical and spiritual. This vulnerability highlights the importance of maintaining both physical and spiritual purity, as the two are deeply interconnected.

OTHER COMMON PARASITES AND THEIR IMPACT ON HUMAN BEHAVIOR

While *Toxoplasma gondii* is one of the most well-known parasites capable of manipulating behavior, it is by no means the only one. Other parasites have been shown to influence their hosts in similarly disturbing ways, affecting everything from mood and decision-making to sexual behavior and social interactions.

ASCARIS LUMBRICOIDES

Overview: *Ascaris lumbricoides* is a type of roundworm that infects the intestines of humans and is one of the most common parasitic infections worldwide. While primarily associated with physical symptoms like malnutrition and gastrointestinal discomfort, *A. lumbricoides* can also affect mental and emotional well-being.

Impact on Cognitive Function: Chronic infections with *A. lumbricoides* can lead to cognitive impairments, particularly in children. These impairments may result from the parasite's depletion of essential nutrients, leading to developmental delays and reduced intellectual functioning. This impact on cognitive function can hinder educational attainment and social development, perpetuating cycles of poverty and poor health.

Behavioral Effects: In addition to cognitive impairments, *A. lumbricoides* infection has been linked to mood disorders such as depression and anxiety. The chronic stress of living with a parasitic infection can lead to emotional instability, irritability, and a sense of hopelessness. These behavioral changes can further isolate individuals from their communities, exacerbating the social and psychological impact of the infection.

TAENIA SOLIUM (PORK TAPEWORM)

Overview: *Taenia solium*, commonly known as the pork tapeworm, can cause a range of health issues in humans, particularly when its larvae migrate to the brain, leading to a condition known as neurocysticercosis. This condition can have severe neurological and psychological effects.

Neurological Impact: Neurocysticercosis is a major cause of epilepsy in regions where *T. solium* is prevalent. The presence of cysts in the brain can lead to seizures, headaches, and other neurological symptoms. These physical manifestations are often accompanied by changes in behavior, including confusion, paranoia, and psychosis.

Spiritual and Psychological Consequences: The neurological impact of *T. solium* infection can be seen as a form of spiritual assault, where the individual's sense of self is compromised by the parasite's presence in the brain. The resulting behavioral changes can lead to a sense of alienation and loss of identity, further deepening the spiritual and psychological toll of the infection.

ENTAMOEBA HISTOLYTICA

Overview: *Entamoeba histolytica* is a parasitic amoeba that causes amoebiasis, a potentially severe intestinal infection. While primarily affecting the digestive system, severe cases of amoebiasis can lead to abscesses in the liver, lungs, and brain.

Impact on Mental Health: In severe cases where *E. histolytica* spreads to the brain, it can cause neurological symptoms such as confusion, hallucinations, and delirium. These symptoms can be terrifying for the affected individual and their loved ones, leading to a sense of fear and helplessness.

Behavioral Effects: The chronic pain and discomfort associated with amoebiasis can also lead to depression and anxiety. The constant battle with the infection can drain the individual's energy and willpower, leading to a sense of defeat and spiritual exhaustion.

PLASMODIUM SPP. (MALARIA PARASITE)

Overview: The *Plasmodium* species, which causes malaria, is another parasite known to affect human behavior. Malaria is transmitted through the bite of an infected mosquito and primarily affects the liver and red blood cells.

Neurological Impact: Severe malaria can lead to cerebral malaria, a life-threatening condition that affects the brain. Symptoms include seizures, confusion, and coma. Even after recovery, survivors may experience long-term cognitive impairments, including memory loss, difficulty concentrating, and emotional instability.

Behavioral and Social Effects: The chronic fatigue and weakness associated with malaria can lead to social withdrawal and a lack of motivation. In communities where malaria is endemic, the constant threat of illness can create a pervasive sense of fear and fatalism, affecting social cohesion and community morale.

THE BROADER IMPLICATIONS OF PARASITIC INFLUENCE ON MENTAL AND SPIRITUAL HEALTH

The ability of parasites to manipulate human behavior has profound implications for our understanding of health and spirituality. These findings challenge the conventional view of free will and autonomy, suggesting that our thoughts, emotions, and actions may be influenced by unseen forces. This realization has important implications for both individual well-being and society as a whole.

THE EROSION OF AUTONOMY AND FREE WILL

Loss of Control: The manipulation of behavior by parasites represents a fundamental challenge to the concept of free will. If our actions can be influenced by a microscopic organism within our bodies, then our sense of autonomy is compromised. This loss of control can lead to a feeling of powerlessness and spiritual disconnection, as individuals struggle to understand and overcome the influences affecting their behavior.

Spiritual Consequences: From a spiritual perspective, the erosion of free will by parasitic influence can be seen as a form of possession or spiritual hijacking. Just as demonic forces are believed to control individuals and lead them away from their true path, parasites can subtly alter behavior in ways that serve their own interests rather than the well-being of the host. This spiritual hijacking can lead to a sense of alienation from the divine and a loss of spiritual clarity.

THE IMPACT ON MENTAL HEALTH

Mental Disorders and Parasitic Infections: The connection between parasitic infections and mental health disorders is an area of growing interest in both scientific and spiritual communities. Parasites like *T. gondii* have been linked to conditions such as schizophrenia, bipolar disorder, and depression, raising questions about the role of biological factors in mental illness. These findings suggest that addressing parasitic infections may be an important component of treating and preventing mental health disorders.

The Stigma of Parasitic Influence: The association between parasites and mental health disorders can also contribute to stigma and social isolation. Individuals affected by parasitic infections may be seen as unclean or spiritually impure, leading to discrimination and exclusion from their communities. This stigma can exacerbate the psychological and spiritual impact of the infection, creating a vicious cycle of suffering and marginalization.

PARASITES AND SUICIDAL IDEATION: THE HIDDEN INFLUENCE ON MENTAL HEALTH

THE DARK INFLUENCE OF PARASITES ON MOOD AND BEHAVIOR

Parasites are not just physical invaders; they are also insidious influencers of mental and emotional well-being. While much of the public's understanding of parasites focuses on physical symptoms, the psychological and neurological impacts are often overlooked. These microorganisms can manipulate the brain's chemistry, leading to a wide range of mental health issues, including depression, anxiety, and even suicidal ideation.

One of the most well-known parasites that affect human behavior is *Toxoplasma gondii*. This parasite is notorious for its ability to alter the behavior of its host, and studies have shown a correlation between *T. gondii* infection and increased rates of suicide, particularly in women. The parasite is believed to affect neurotransmitter levels in the brain, such as dopamine, which can lead to mood swings, impulsive behavior, and severe depression.

However, *T. gondii* is not the only parasite with this dark influence. Other parasites, such as *Ascaris lumbricoides* (roundworms), *Taenia solium* (tapeworms), and *Plasmodium spp.* (which causes malaria), have also been linked to neurological symptoms, including mood disorders. These parasites can induce chronic inflammation, disrupt normal brain function, and create an environment in the body that contributes to mental health disorders.

PARASITES AND MOOD DISORDERS: A HIDDEN EPIDEMIC

It is not uncommon for individuals suffering from mood disorders to seek treatment for depression, anxiety, or bipolar disorder without ever considering that their symptoms might be caused by parasitic infections. Traditional medical approaches often focus on managing symptoms through medication, which may temporarily alleviate the issue but does not address the root cause. As a result, many people continue to suffer from mood swings, anxiety attacks, and suicidal thoughts without realizing that their mental health issues may be driven by parasites.

Chronic parasitic infections can lead to a constant state of low-grade inflammation in the body, which in turn affects the brain. This inflammation disrupts the production and regulation of key neurotransmitters such as serotonin, dopamine, and GABA, which are critical for mood regulation. The resulting imbalance can manifest as depression, anxiety, irritability, and even psychosis. In severe cases, the feelings of hopelessness and despair can become so overwhelming that individuals may contemplate or attempt suicide.

THE IMPORTANCE OF ADDRESSING PARASITIC INFECTIONS IN MENTAL HEALTH

Given the profound impact that parasites can have on mental health, it is essential to consider parasitic infections as a potential underlying cause of mood disorders. For those experiencing unexplained or treatment-resistant depression, anxiety, or suicidal ideation, it may be beneficial to undergo testing for parasites and other hidden infections. Ayurvedic practices, with their focus on detoxification and purification, offer effective ways to address these infections and restore balance to both the body and mind.

Ayurvedic herbs like Neem, Vidanga, and Turmeric, as well as Panchakarma therapies, can help eliminate parasites and reduce the inflammation they cause. Additionally, adopting a Sattvik lifestyle, which emphasizes a clean diet, regular fasting, and spiritual practices, can strengthen the body's defenses against parasitic infections and support mental and emotional well-being.

THE SOCIAL AND CULTURAL IMPLICATIONS

Public Health and Parasitic Infections: The widespread prevalence of parasitic infections has significant implications for public health, particularly in regions where access to clean water, sanitation, and healthcare is limited. Addressing these infections requires a holistic approach that considers not only the biological aspects of the disease but also the social, cultural, and spiritual factors that influence health and well-being.

Cultural Beliefs and Health Practices: Cultural beliefs about parasites and their influence on behavior can shape health practices and public health interventions. In some cultures, traditional healers and spiritual leaders play a central role in diagnosing and treating parasitic infections, using rituals, herbal remedies, and spiritual practices to restore balance and health. Recognizing the value of these traditional approaches can enhance the effectiveness of public health initiatives and promote culturally sensitive care.

NTEGRATING MODERN SCIENCE WITH TRADITIONAL WISDOM

A Holistic Approach to Health: The integration of modern scientific knowledge with traditional spiritual wisdom offers a powerful approach to understanding and addressing the impact of parasites on human behavior. By combining medical treatments with spiritual practices such as fasting, prayer, and purification rituals, individuals can protect themselves from both the physical and spiritual aspects of parasitic influence.

Empowerment Through Knowledge: Educating individuals and communities about the connection between parasites and behavior can empower them to take control of their health and well-being. By understanding the ways in which parasites can manipulate behavior, individuals can make informed choices about their diet, hygiene, and spiritual practices, reducing their vulnerability to parasitic influences and strengthening their spiritual sovereignty.

The ability of parasites to manipulate human behavior challenges our understanding of autonomy, free will, and the nature of spiritual influence. Parasites like *Toxoplasma gondii*, *Ascaris lumbricoides*, and *Taenia solium* can alter behavior in ways that serve their own survival, often at the expense of the host's health and well-being. These manipulations have profound implications for mental and spiritual health, raising important questions about the role of biological factors in shaping our thoughts, emotions, and actions.

By exploring the connections between parasites and behavior through both scientific and spiritual lenses, we gain a deeper understanding of the ways in which our health and spiritual well-being are interconnected. This knowledge empowers us to take a holistic approach to health, integrating modern medical treatments with traditional spiritual practices to protect ourselves from the parasitic forces that seek to undermine our autonomy and spiritual clarity.

MEAT PUPPETS: HOW PARASITES CONTROL YOUR BODY, MIND & SPIRIT

In many ancient traditions, the struggle for spiritual sovereignty—the ability to maintain control over one's mind, body, and spirit—is seen as a fundamental aspect of human life. This struggle often involves combating various external and internal forces that seek to undermine this sovereignty. Among these forces, parasites play a unique role, acting as both physical invaders and symbolic representations of demonic influences that weaken the spirit. This chapter explores the connection between parasitic infections and the erosion of spiritual sovereignty, drawing parallels between ancient concepts of demonic possession and the modern understanding of parasitic influence on behavior and health.

PARASITES, DEMONS, AND THE WEAKENING OF SPIRITUAL SOVEREIGNTY

THE SPIRITUAL AND PHYSICAL CONSEQUENCES OF PARASITIC INFECTION

Parasites, by their very nature, thrive at the expense of their hosts. They consume the host's nutrients, compromise immune function, and in many cases, manipulate the host's behavior to ensure their own survival. Beyond these physical effects, parasites can also have profound spiritual consequences, leading to a weakening of the individual's connection to the divine and a loss of control over their own life.

THE PHYSICAL TOLL OF PARASITIC INFECTIONS

Nutrient Depletion and Immune Suppression: Parasites such as *Ascaris lumbricoides* and *Taenia solium* deplete the body of essential nutrients, leading to malnutrition, fatigue, and weakened immunity. This physical toll can leave individuals more vulnerable to other infections and diseases, creating a cycle of illness that is difficult to break.

Chronic Illness and Mental Health: The physical burden of parasitic infections can also have a significant impact on mental health. Chronic pain, fatigue, and the psychological stress of living with a persistent infection can lead to depression, anxiety, and other mental health disorders. These conditions further erode the individual's ability to maintain spiritual clarity and resilience.

THE EROSION OF SPIRITUAL SOVEREIGNTY

Loss of Autonomy: Parasitic infections can lead to a loss of autonomy, both physically and spiritually. As the parasite takes control of the host's body, manipulating behavior and depleting resources, the individual may feel increasingly powerless and disconnected from their true self. This loss of autonomy is mirrored on a spiritual level, where the individual may struggle to maintain a sense of purpose and direction in life.

Spiritual Disconnection: The presence of parasites in the body can create a sense of spiritual disconnection, as the individual becomes preoccupied with physical symptoms and the emotional toll of illness. This disconnection can lead to feelings of isolation, hopelessness, and a loss of faith, further weakening the individual's spiritual sovereignty.

Symbolic Possession: In many cultures, parasitic infections are seen as a form of symbolic possession, where the individual is "possessed" by the parasite and its influence. This concept parallels ancient beliefs in demonic possession, where negative spiritual forces take control of the individual's mind and body, leading them away from their true path.

THE PARALLELS BETWEEN PARASITES AND DEMONIC POSSESSION

Manipulation of Behavior: Just as demonic forces are believed to manipulate individuals to act against their better judgment, parasites manipulate their hosts to behave in ways that benefit the parasite. This manipulation can lead to risky behaviors, impaired judgment, and a loss of self-control, all of which undermine spiritual sovereignty.

Erosion of Free Will: The erosion of free will is a central theme in both parasitic infections and demonic possession. In both cases, the individual's ability to make conscious, autonomous decisions is compromised, leading to a sense of powerlessness and spiritual disorientation. This loss of free will is a key factor in the weakening of spiritual sovereignty.

Spiritual Contamination: In many traditions, parasites are seen as agents of spiritual contamination, bringing impurity and corruption into the body. This contamination can manifest as physical illness, moral decay, or a loss of spiritual clarity, all of which contribute to the erosion of spiritual sovereignty.

AYURVEDIC AND HINDU SOLUTIONS FOR RECLAIMING SPIRITUAL SOVEREIGNTY

In the face of these challenges, Ayurveda and Hindu practices offer powerful tools for reclaiming spiritual sovereignty and protecting against parasitic influences. These practices emphasize the importance of purity, balance, and spiritual discipline in maintaining control over one's mind, body, and spirit.

AYURVEDIC REMEDIES FOR PARASITES

Detoxification and Cleansing: Ayurveda places a strong emphasis on detoxification and cleansing as a means of removing parasites and restoring balance to the body. Panchakarma, a traditional Ayurvedic detoxification therapy, involves a series of treatments such as Vamana (therapeutic vomiting), Virechana (therapeutic purgation), and Basti (medicated enemas) that are designed to eliminate toxins and parasites from the body. These treatments help to restore physical health and enhance spiritual clarity by purging the body of impurities.

Herbal Remedies: Ayurveda also utilizes a wide range of herbal remedies to combat parasitic infections and strengthen the body's defenses. Herbs such as neem, vidanga, and turmeric are known for their antiparasitic properties and are commonly used in Ayurvedic treatments. These herbs not only help to eliminate parasites but also support the immune system and promote overall health, making the body less susceptible to parasitic influences.

Balancing the Doshas: In Ayurveda, health is seen as a state of balance between the three doshas—Vata, Pitta, and Kapha. Imbalances in these doshas can create an environment in which parasites thrive. Ayurvedic treatments aim to restore this balance through diet, lifestyle changes, and herbal remedies, thereby reducing the risk of parasitic infections and enhancing spiritual sovereignty.

HINDU PRACTICES FOR SPIRITUAL PROTECTION

Fasting as a Spiritual Discipline: Fasting is a central practice in Hinduism, used not only for physical purification but also for spiritual protection. Regular fasting helps to cleanse the body of toxins and parasites, while also strengthening the mind and spirit. By denying the physical body and focusing on spiritual practices, individuals can enhance their spiritual resilience and maintain control over their thoughts and actions. Fasting also helps to cultivate self-discipline and mindfulness, which are essential for maintaining spiritual sovereignty.

Mantras and Meditation: Hinduism emphasizes the use of mantras and meditation as tools for protecting against negative influences and strengthening spiritual sovereignty. Mantras such as the Mahamrityunjaya Mantra, which is dedicated to Lord Shiva and is believed to protect against death and disease, can be used to create a protective shield around the individual. Meditation practices, such as focusing on the third eye (Ajna Chakra), help to enhance spiritual awareness and maintain a connection to the divine.

Rituals and Offerings: Hindu rituals and offerings play a crucial role in maintaining spiritual sovereignty. Rituals such as Agnihotra (fire sacrifice) are performed to purify the environment and protect against negative influences, including parasitic forces. Offerings made to deities, such as food, flowers, and incense, help to cultivate a relationship with the divine and strengthen spiritual protection. These rituals not only protect against parasitic influences but also reinforce the individual's connection to their spiritual path.

THE SATTVIK LIFESTYLE: A HOLISTIC APPROACH TO SPIRITUAL SOVEREIGNTY

Purity in Diet and Lifestyle: The sattvik lifestyle, which emphasizes purity in diet and lifestyle, is designed to support both physical and spiritual health. By following a sattvik diet—one that is vegetarian, fresh, and balanced—individuals can maintain a strong digestive fire (Agni) and reduce the risk of parasitic infections. The sattvik lifestyle also emphasizes cleanliness, moderation, and mindfulness in all aspects of life, helping to cultivate an environment in which parasites cannot thrive.

Regular Spiritual Practice: Regular spiritual practice is a key component of the sattvik lifestyle. This includes daily rituals, prayer, meditation, and the chanting of mantras. These practices help to maintain spiritual clarity, protect against negative influences, and strengthen the individual's connection to the divine. By incorporating these practices into daily life, individuals can maintain spiritual sovereignty and resist the influence of parasitic forces.

Harmony with Nature: The sattvik lifestyle also promotes harmony with nature, recognizing the interconnectedness of all living beings. This holistic approach encourages individuals to live in balance with their environment, respecting the natural world and its cycles. By cultivating a deep connection with nature, individuals can enhance their spiritual resilience and protect against the disruptive influences of parasites and other negative forces.

THE ROLE OF FASTING IN MAINTAINING SPIRITUAL SOVEREIGNTY

Fasting is a practice that has been revered across cultures and religions for its powerful effects on both physical and spiritual health. In Hinduism, fasting is not merely a dietary practice but a profound spiritual discipline that helps maintain spiritual sovereignty and protect against parasitic influences.

THE SPIRITUAL POWER OF FASTING

Purification of the Body and Soul: Fasting is seen as a means of purifying both the body and the soul. By abstaining from food, the body enters a state of detoxification, eliminating toxins and parasites that may have accumulated over time. This physical purification is mirrored by a spiritual purification, as fasting helps to clear the mind and focus on spiritual practices. The act of fasting is a form of self-discipline that strengthens the will and enhances spiritual resilience.

Connection to the Divine: Fasting is also a way to deepen one's connection to the divine. By denying the physical body, individuals can focus more fully on their spiritual practices, such as prayer, meditation, and the chanting of mantras. This heightened spiritual focus helps to strengthen the individual's connection to their higher self and the divine, reinforcing their spiritual sovereignty.

Protection Against Negative Influences: Fasting is believed to protect against negative influences, both physical and spiritual. By purifying the body and mind, fasting creates a protective shield that guards against parasitic forces and other negative entities. This protection is enhanced by the spiritual practices that accompany fasting, such as prayer and meditation, which help to strengthen the individual's spiritual defenses.

THE REMOVAL OF FASTING FROM MODERN TRADITIONS

Diminished Spiritual Discipline: In many modern religious traditions, particularly within Christianity, the practice of fasting has been diminished or even removed altogether. This shift has significant implications for spiritual sovereignty, as the absence of fasting weakens the individual's ability to resist negative influences and maintain spiritual clarity. The removal of fasting from religious practice can be seen as a loss of a vital tool for spiritual protection and self-discipline.

Vulnerability to Parasitic Influences: The decline of fasting in modern religious traditions has left many individuals more vulnerable to parasitic influences. Without the regular practice of fasting, the body and mind become more susceptible to the accumulation of toxins and parasites, leading to physical and spiritual decay. This vulnerability is compounded by the loss of spiritual discipline and focus, making it more difficult for individuals to maintain control over their own lives.

The Contrast with Hindu Traditions: In contrast, fasting remains a central practice in Hinduism, where it is used to maintain both physical and spiritual health. The continued emphasis on fasting in Hindu culture has helped its followers maintain spiritual sovereignty and resist the influence of parasitic forces. This commitment to regular purification and self-discipline serves as a powerful example of how traditional practices can protect against the challenges of modern life.

FASTING AND THE PRESERVATION OF SPIRITUAL SOVEREIGNTY

A Holistic Approach to Health: Fasting, when combined with other spiritual practices such as prayer, meditation, and ritual, offers a holistic approach to maintaining spiritual sovereignty. By addressing both the physical and spiritual aspects of health, fasting helps individuals maintain control over their thoughts, actions, and spiritual path. This holistic approach recognizes the interconnectedness of body, mind, and spirit, ensuring that all aspects of the individual are protected and nurtured.

The Role of the Sattvik Lifestyle: The sattvik lifestyle, with its emphasis on purity, balance, and spiritual discipline, provides a strong foundation for fasting and other spiritual practices. By following a sattvik lifestyle, individuals can maintain a state of physical and spiritual purity that supports fasting and enhances its benefits. This lifestyle promotes harmony with nature, respect for the body, and a deep connection to the divine, all of which are essential for preserving spiritual sovereignty.

Parasites, both physical and symbolic, pose a significant threat to spiritual sovereignty. By manipulating behavior, depleting resources, and eroding free will, these parasitic forces weaken the individual's connection to their true self and the divine. The parallels between parasitic infections and demonic possession highlight the profound spiritual consequences of losing control over one's mind, body, and spirit.

In response to these challenges, Ayurveda and Hindu practices offer powerful tools for reclaiming spiritual sovereignty and protecting against parasitic influences. Through detoxification, herbal remedies, fasting, and regular spiritual practice, individuals can purify their bodies and minds, strengthen their spiritual defenses, and maintain control over their own lives.

By embracing a holistic approach to health—one that integrates physical, mental, and spiritual well-being—we can protect ourselves from the parasitic forces that seek to undermine our autonomy and spiritual clarity. The practices of fasting, meditation, and the sattvik lifestyle offer a path to preserving spiritual sovereignty, ensuring that we remain connected to our true selves and the divine.

PART 5

RECLAIMING CONTROL: A HOLISTIC APPROACH TO HEALTH AND SPIRITUALITY

The journey toward reclaiming spiritual sovereignty and protecting oneself from parasitic influences requires more than just awareness and intention; it demands practical, actionable steps rooted in ancient wisdom and holistic health practices. Ayurveda, the traditional system of medicine from India, offers a comprehensive approach to detoxification and fasting that not only cleanses the body of physical impurities but also fortifies the spirit. This chapter delves into the Ayurvedic methods for detoxifying the body, the spiritual significance of fasting, and the enduring wisdom of Hindu practices in maintaining physical and spiritual health.

AYURVEDIC DETOXIFICATION AND FASTING

THE ROLE OF PANCHAKARMA IN CLEANSING PARASITES

Panchakarma is one of the most revered detoxification and purification therapies in Ayurveda. It is a five-fold treatment that targets the removal of deep-seated toxins (Ama) from the body, rejuvenates the organs, and restores balance to the doshas. Panchakarma is particularly effective in eliminating parasites and other harmful entities that disrupt the body's natural harmony.

THE PRINCIPLES OF PANCHAKARMA

Detoxification and Rejuvenation: Panchakarma is designed to cleanse the body at the cellular level, removing toxins that accumulate from poor diet, environmental pollutants, stress, and parasitic infections. It also aims to rejuvenate the body's tissues (Dhatus) and strengthen the immune system, ensuring long-term health and vitality.

Restoring Dosha Balance: The three doshas—Vata, Pitta, and Kapha—are the fundamental energies that govern the body's functions. Imbalances in these doshas can create an environment in which parasites thrive. Panchakarma treatments are customized to restore balance to the doshas, promoting overall health and reducing susceptibility to parasitic infections.

THE FIVE THERAPIES OF PANCHAKARMA

Vamana (Therapeutic Vomiting): Vamana is a treatment that induces vomiting to expel excess Kapha dosha from the body. This therapy is particularly effective in removing mucus, toxins, and parasites from the stomach and respiratory tract. By clearing these channels, Vamana helps to restore balance and prevent the conditions that allow parasites to thrive.

Virechana (Therapeutic Purgation): Virechana involves the administration of purgative substances to cleanse the intestines and liver, removing excess Pitta dosha. This treatment is effective in eliminating toxins and parasites from the digestive system, promoting healthy digestion and preventing the buildup of harmful entities.

Basti (Medicated Enemas): Basti is a powerful therapy that involves the administration of herbal enemas to cleanse the colon and balance Vata dosha. Basti is particularly effective in removing parasites from the lower digestive tract, as well as in rejuvenating the body's tissues and improving overall health.

Nasya (Nasal Administration): Nasya involves the administration of medicated oils or powders through the nostrils to clear the sinuses and respiratory tract. This treatment helps to remove toxins and parasites from the head and neck region, promoting clarity of mind and protecting against infections.

Raktamokshana (Bloodletting): Raktamokshana is a therapeutic bloodletting procedure used to purify the blood and remove toxins from the circulatory system. While less commonly practiced today, this therapy was traditionally used to treat conditions caused by excess Pitta dosha and to expel parasites that reside in the blood.

THE SPIRITUAL BENEFITS OF PANCHAKARMA

Cleansing the Mind and Spirit: Panchakarma is not only a physical detoxification process but also a spiritual cleansing. By removing toxins and parasites from the body, Panchakarma helps to clear the mind, enhance spiritual awareness, and strengthen the connection to the divine. This purification process is essential for maintaining spiritual sovereignty and resisting negative influences.

Rejuvenation and Renewal: The rejuvenating effects of Panchakarma extend beyond the physical body to the mind and spirit. After completing Panchakarma, individuals often experience a sense of renewal, increased vitality, and enhanced spiritual clarity. This rejuvenation supports long-term health and well-being, providing a strong foundation for spiritual growth.

FASTING IN HINDUISM AND AYURVEDA

Fasting, or *Upavasa*, is a profound spiritual discipline that has been practiced in Hinduism for thousands of years. It is not merely an act of abstaining from food but a holistic practice that involves physical, mental, and spiritual purification. In Ayurveda, fasting is recognized as a powerful tool for detoxification, healing, and maintaining balance in the body and mind.

THE SPIRITUAL SIGNIFICANCE OF FASTING

Connection to the Divine: Fasting is seen as a means of drawing closer to the divine by denying the physical body and focusing on spiritual practices. By abstaining from food, individuals create space for spiritual reflection, prayer, and meditation. This heightened spiritual focus helps to strengthen the connection to the divine and enhance spiritual sovereignty.

Purification and Self-Discipline: Fasting is also a form of self-discipline that purifies both the body and the mind. By controlling the urges of the physical body, individuals cultivate greater self-control and mindfulness, which are essential for spiritual growth. The act of fasting helps to cleanse the body of toxins and parasites, while also clearing the mind of distractions and negative thoughts.

THE AYURVEDIC PERSPECTIVE ON FASTING

Types of Fasting: Ayurveda recognizes different types of fasting, depending on the individual's constitution (Prakriti) and health condition. These range from complete fasting (Nirahara) to partial fasting, where certain foods or meals are skipped. The type and duration of fasting are tailored to the individual's needs, ensuring that the practice is both effective and safe.

Fasting and Agni (Digestive Fire): Ayurveda emphasizes the importance of Agni, or digestive fire, in maintaining health. When Agni is strong, the body can efficiently digest food, absorb nutrients, and eliminate waste. Fasting helps to strengthen Agni by giving the digestive system a rest and allowing it to reset. This enhanced digestive capacity not only improves overall health but also creates an inhospitable environment for parasites.

Detoxification and Healing: Fasting is a powerful method of detoxification in Ayurveda. By abstaining from food, the body can focus on eliminating accumulated toxins (Ama) that contribute to disease and imbalance. Fasting helps to clear the channels (Srotas) of the body, improving circulation, digestion, and the elimination of waste. This detoxification process is particularly effective in removing parasites and other harmful entities from the body.

THE ROLE OF FASTING IN MAINTAINING SPIRITUAL AND PHYSICAL HEALTH

Regular Fasting Practices: In Hinduism, fasting is a regular practice that is observed on specific days of the week, during religious festivals, or on particular lunar days such as Ekadashi and Purnima. These fasts serve not only as spiritual disciplines but also as opportunities for physical detoxification and rejuvenation. By incorporating regular fasting into their lives, individuals can maintain physical and spiritual health, reducing their vulnerability to parasitic influences.

Fasting and Mental Clarity: One of the key benefits of fasting is its impact on mental clarity and focus. By giving the digestive system a rest, fasting frees up energy that can be redirected to the brain and nervous system. This enhanced mental clarity supports spiritual practices such as meditation and prayer, allowing individuals to deepen their spiritual connection and maintain spiritual sovereignty.

Fasting as a Form of Resistance: In a world where the consumption of unhealthy, processed foods is prevalent, fasting can be seen as a form of resistance. By choosing to fast, individuals reject the temptations of the material world and reaffirm their commitment to spiritual purity and self-discipline. This act of resistance strengthens spiritual sovereignty and protects against the negative influences of parasitic forces.

INCORPORATING SALT AND HERBS IN DETOXIFICATION

In addition to fasting and Panchakarma, Ayurveda emphasizes the use of salt and specific herbs to create an inhospitable environment for parasites and support overall health. These natural remedies have been used for centuries to purify the body, enhance digestion, and protect against infections.

THE PURIFYING POWER OF SALT

Salt in Ayurvedic Medicine: Salt, particularly natural sea salt, is considered a purifying substance in Ayurveda. It is used in various Ayurvedic treatments to cleanse the body and enhance the effectiveness of other therapies. Salt helps to balance the doshas, improve digestion, and eliminate toxins, making it an essential component of detoxification practices.

Salt and Parasite Control: Salt is known for its antimicrobial properties, making it effective in controlling parasites and other harmful organisms. In Ayurveda, salt is often added to herbal preparations and used in detoxification therapies to enhance their potency. Regular consumption of a moderate amount of natural sea salt can support digestive health and protect against parasitic infections.

Spiritual Significance of Salt: Beyond its physical benefits, salt also holds spiritual significance in many cultures. In Hinduism, salt is used in rituals to purify spaces and objects, as well as to protect against negative energies. This dual role of salt as both a physical and spiritual purifying agent highlights its importance in maintaining health and spiritual sovereignty.

THE USE OF AYURVEDIC HERBS FOR PARASITE ELIMINATION

Neem (*Azadirachta indica*): Neem is one of the most powerful antiparasitic herbs in Ayurveda. It has strong antimicrobial properties and is used to cleanse the blood, improve digestion, and eliminate parasites from the body. Neem is often taken as a powder, capsule, or in the form of a decoction, and can be combined with other herbs to enhance its effectiveness.

Vidanga (*Embelia ribes*): Vidanga is another potent antiparasitic herb used in Ayurveda. It is particularly effective against intestinal worms and is often included in herbal formulations designed to cleanse the digestive system. Vidanga also helps to strengthen Agni, ensuring that the digestive system remains robust and capable of resisting parasitic infections.

Turmeric (*Curcuma longa*): Turmeric is renowned for its anti-inflammatory and antimicrobial properties. In Ayurveda, it is used to purify the blood, support liver function, and protect against infections, including those caused by parasites. Turmeric can be consumed as a spice, in herbal preparations, or as a supplement, making it a versatile tool in maintaining health and spiritual clarity.

Triphala: Triphala is a traditional Ayurvedic formulation consisting of three fruits—Amalaki, Bibhitaki, and Haritaki. It is a powerful detoxifier and rejuvenator, known for its ability to cleanse the digestive system, eliminate toxins, and support overall health. Triphala is often used in Panchakarma and other detoxification therapies to enhance their effectiveness and promote long-term health.

THE INTEGRATION OF FASTING AND DETOXIFICATION INTO MODERN LIFE

While the practices of Panchakarma, fasting, and the use of Ayurvedic herbs are rooted in ancient wisdom, they remain highly relevant in today's world. Modern lifestyles, with their exposure to processed foods, environmental toxins, and stress, create a fertile ground for parasites and other negative influences. By integrating these traditional practices into daily life, individuals can protect themselves from these challenges and maintain their spiritual sovereignty.

PRACTICAL TIPS FOR INCORPORATING FASTING AND DETOXIFICATION

Start Small: If you are new to fasting or Ayurvedic detoxification, it is important to start small and gradually build up your practice. Begin with short fasts, such as skipping a meal or fasting for half a day, and slowly increase the duration as your body becomes accustomed to the practice. Similarly, start with gentle detoxification therapies, such as taking Triphala or incorporating detoxifying herbs into your diet, before attempting more intensive treatments like Panchakarma.

Listen to Your Body: Fasting and detoxification should be tailored to your individual needs and constitution. Pay attention to how your body responds to these practices and adjust them accordingly. If you experience any discomfort or adverse effects, consult with an Ayurvedic practitioner who can guide you in finding the right approach for your unique constitution.

Incorporate Rituals: To enhance the spiritual benefits of fasting and detoxification, consider incorporating rituals such as prayer, meditation, and the chanting of mantras into your practice. These rituals help to focus the mind, strengthen your spiritual connection, and create a protective environment that supports your healing journey.

THE SATTVIK LIFESTYLE AS A FOUNDATION FOR HEALTH

Maintain a Balanced Diet: The sattvik lifestyle emphasizes the importance of a balanced diet that supports physical, mental, and spiritual health. Focus on consuming fresh, whole foods that are easy to digest and free from toxins. Avoid processed foods, excessive sugar, and heavy, tamasic foods that can disrupt your digestion and create an environment in which parasites thrive.

Practice Regular Cleansing: Regular cleansing is a key component of the sattvik lifestyle. This can include daily practices such as oil pulling, dry brushing, and tongue scraping, as well as seasonal detoxification therapies like Panchakarma. These practices help to remove toxins, support digestion, and maintain overall health.

Embrace Spiritual Practices: The sattvik lifestyle also includes regular spiritual practices that help to maintain spiritual sovereignty. These can include daily rituals, prayer, meditation, and the chanting of mantras. By incorporating these practices into your daily routine, you can protect yourself from negative influences and cultivate a deep connection with the divine.

The practices of Ayurvedic detoxification and fasting offer powerful tools for maintaining both physical and spiritual health. By cleansing the body of toxins and parasites, these practices help to restore balance, enhance spiritual clarity, and protect against negative influences. The integration of these ancient practices into modern life provides a holistic approach to health that addresses the interconnectedness of body, mind, and spirit.

Fasting, in particular, serves as a profound spiritual discipline that strengthens self-discipline, enhances mental clarity, and deepens the connection to the divine. Combined with the use of Ayurvedic herbs and the principles of the sattvik lifestyle, fasting and detoxification offer a comprehensive approach to maintaining spiritual sovereignty and resisting the influence of parasitic forces.

As you embark on this journey of purification and healing, remember that the path to spiritual sovereignty is a continuous process of self-care, discipline, and mindfulness. By embracing these practices, you can protect yourself from the challenges of modern life and cultivate a state of health and well-being that supports your spiritual growth and connection to the divine.

In the pursuit of spiritual sovereignty, the ancient wisdom of Hindu practices offers a rich tapestry of rituals, mantras, and meditations that serve to protect the spirit, purify the body, and strengthen the connection to the divine. These practices are not merely ceremonial; they are deeply rooted in a philosophy that recognizes the interconnectedness of the physical and spiritual realms. This chapter explores the power of Hindu rituals, mantras, and daily spiritual practices in reclaiming and maintaining spiritual sovereignty, with a focus on how these practices protect against the parasitic influences that seek to undermine our autonomy.

RECLAIMING SPIRITUAL SOVEREIGNTY THROUGH HINDU PRACTICES

SPIRITUAL PRACTICES FOR PROTECTION

The journey toward spiritual sovereignty is one of both inner transformation and external protection. Hindu practices offer a range of tools to shield the individual from negative influences, whether they are physical, emotional, or spiritual. These practices are designed to purify the body and mind, create a protective aura, and fortify the individual's spiritual defenses.

THE ROLE OF RITUALS IN SPIRITUAL PROTECTION

Agnihotra (Fire Ritual): Agnihotra is a Vedic fire ritual performed at sunrise and sunset. This practice involves offering specific substances into a sacred fire while chanting mantras, creating an environment that is both physically and spiritually purifying. The fire is believed to consume impurities, including negative energies and parasitic influences, both within the individual and in the surrounding environment. Agnihotra not only purifies the air and atmosphere but also strengthens the individual's connection to the divine, creating a protective barrier against negative forces.

Abhishekam (Ritual Bathing of Deities): Abhishekam is a ritual in which deities are bathed in sacred substances such as milk, honey, yogurt, and water. This act of devotion is believed to purify both the deity and the devotee, removing negative energies and enhancing spiritual protection. The substances used in Abhishekam are symbolic of various aspects of life and are believed to carry purifying properties that protect against spiritual contamination.

Puja (Worship): Puja is a daily ritual of offering flowers, food, incense, and prayers to deities. This practice helps to cultivate a deep connection with the divine and invite blessings of protection, health, and spiritual strength. Puja is a way of acknowledging the divine presence in one's life and seeking its protection against all forms of negativity, including parasitic influences.

THE POWER OF MANTRAS IN CREATING A PROTECTIVE SHIELD

Mahamrityunjaya Mantra: The Mahamrityunjaya Mantra is one of the most powerful mantras in Hinduism, dedicated to Lord Shiva. It is believed to protect against untimely death, disease, and negative influences. Chanting this mantra regularly creates a protective shield around the individual, guarding against physical and spiritual harm. The vibrations of the mantra resonate within the body, purifying the mind and spirit, and fortifying the individual's spiritual defenses.

Gayatri Mantra: The Gayatri Mantra is a revered Vedic prayer that invokes the divine light of the sun to illuminate the mind and spirit. It is chanted to remove ignorance, dispel darkness, and protect against negative influences. The regular chanting of the Gayatri Mantra is believed to strengthen the mind, enhance spiritual clarity, and protect against parasitic forces that seek to cloud judgment and weaken spiritual sovereignty.

Durga Mantra: The Durga Mantra is dedicated to Goddess Durga, the embodiment of divine strength and protection. Chanting this mantra invokes the goddess's power to remove obstacles, protect against evil, and destroy negative forces. The Durga Mantra is particularly effective in combating spiritual attacks and maintaining spiritual sovereignty in the face of adversity.

MEDITATION AND VISUALIZATION FOR SPIRITUAL SOVEREIGNTY

Ajna Chakra Meditation: The Ajna Chakra, or third eye, is associated with intuition, spiritual insight, and inner vision. Meditating on the Ajna Chakra helps to activate and balance this energy center, enhancing spiritual awareness and protection. Through focused meditation on the third eye, individuals can strengthen their spiritual sovereignty, gaining clarity and insight into the forces that influence their lives. This practice helps to cultivate a strong, protective aura that guards against parasitic influences.

Protective Visualization Techniques: Visualization is a powerful tool in spiritual practice, allowing individuals to mentally create protective barriers around themselves. One effective technique is to visualize oneself surrounded by a sphere of white or golden light, representing divine protection. This light forms an impenetrable shield that repels negative energies, parasites, and other harmful influences. Regular practice of protective visualization strengthens spiritual sovereignty and enhances the individual's ability to resist negative forces.

DAILY SPIRITUAL PRACTICES FOR MAINTAINING HEALTH AND SOVEREIGNTY

Sadhana (Daily Spiritual Practice): Sadhana refers to the disciplined practice of spiritual activities, performed daily with dedication and intention. This can include rituals, prayer, mantra chanting, meditation, and self-study (Svadhyaya). Regular Sadhana helps to maintain spiritual sovereignty by keeping the mind focused, the body purified, and the spirit connected to the divine. It is through consistent Sadhana that individuals build spiritual resilience and fortify themselves against the challenges of life, including parasitic influences.

Japa (Mantra Repetition): Japa is the practice of repeating a mantra or divine name, often using a mala (prayer beads) to keep count. This practice helps to focus the mind, purify thoughts, and create a vibration of protection around the individual. The repetition of a sacred mantra or name invokes divine energy, creating a powerful defense against negative influences and strengthening spiritual sovereignty.

Aarti (Ceremonial Light Offering): Aarti is the offering of light, usually in the form of a lit lamp or candle, to the deity. This ritual symbolizes the removal of darkness and ignorance, as well as the offering of one's inner light to the divine. Performing Aarti daily, especially at dawn and dusk, helps to purify the mind and environment, dispelling negativity and enhancing spiritual protection.

THE POWER OF MANTRAS AND RITUALS

Mantras and rituals form the core of Hindu spiritual practice, serving as potent tools for invoking divine protection, purifying the body and mind, and maintaining spiritual sovereignty. These practices are deeply embedded in the Hindu tradition, with each mantra and ritual carrying specific vibrations and intentions that align the individual with higher spiritual forces.

THE SIGNIFICANCE OF MANTRAS IN HINDUISM

Vibrational Healing: Mantras are composed of sacred syllables and sounds that carry specific vibrational frequencies. These vibrations resonate within the body and mind, creating a harmonizing effect that purifies and protects. Chanting mantras regularly helps to align the individual's energy with the divine, creating a powerful defense against negative influences, including parasites.

Mantras as Tools for Transformation: Beyond protection, mantras are also tools for spiritual transformation. They help to focus the mind, cultivate inner peace, and awaken higher consciousness. Through the regular practice of mantra chanting, individuals can transform their inner state, clearing away negativity and enhancing spiritual clarity. This transformation strengthens spiritual sovereignty, empowering individuals to resist parasitic influences and maintain control over their lives.

THE ROLE OF RITUALS IN PURIFICATION AND PROTECTION

Rituals as Expressions of Devotion: Hindu rituals are acts of devotion that create a sacred space in which the divine is honored and invoked. These rituals are performed with specific intentions, such as purification, protection, and the removal of obstacles. By participating in these rituals, individuals align themselves with divine energies, creating a protective shield that guards against negative forces.

Fire Rituals (Agnihotra and Havan): Fire rituals, such as Agnihotra and Havan, are particularly powerful in Hinduism. The sacred fire is believed to have the ability to consume impurities, both physical and spiritual, transforming them into pure energy. These rituals are performed to purify the environment, protect against negative influences, and strengthen the connection to the divine. The smoke from the fire carries the prayers and offerings to the heavens, creating a bridge between the physical and spiritual realms.

Purification Rituals: Purification rituals, such as Abhishekam and the sprinkling of holy water, are performed to cleanse the body, mind, and environment of negative energies. These rituals are often accompanied by the chanting of mantras and the offering of flowers, incense, and other sacred substances. Through these acts of purification, individuals can remove the influences of parasitic forces and restore spiritual clarity and strength.

RECLAIMING SPIRITUAL SOVEREIGNTY THROUGH HINDU PRACTICES

The journey of reclaiming spiritual sovereignty is an ongoing process that requires dedication, mindfulness, and a deep connection to the divine. Hindu practices offer a comprehensive approach to achieving and maintaining this sovereignty, integrating physical, mental, and spiritual disciplines that protect against parasitic influences and support overall well-being.

THE IMPORTANCE OF REGULAR SPIRITUAL PRACTICE

Consistency and Discipline: Regular spiritual practice is essential for maintaining spiritual sovereignty. By dedicating time each day to rituals, mantra chanting, meditation, and prayer, individuals create a strong foundation for spiritual growth and protection. Consistency in practice builds spiritual resilience, enabling individuals to withstand challenges and resist negative influences.

Cultivating Inner Strength: Spiritual practices such as meditation, mantra chanting, and rituals help to cultivate inner strength and resilience. This inner strength is crucial for maintaining spiritual sovereignty, as it allows individuals to remain centered and focused even in the face of adversity. By developing this inner strength, individuals can resist the influence of parasitic forces and maintain control over their thoughts, actions, and spiritual path.

THE ROLE OF COMMUNITY IN SPIRITUAL SOVEREIGNTY

Satsang (Spiritual Community): Being part of a spiritual community, or Satsang, provides support, encouragement, and accountability in one's spiritual journey. In Hinduism, Satsang is valued as a source of collective spiritual energy, where individuals come together to share knowledge, chant mantras, and participate in rituals. The collective energy of the community strengthens each individual's spiritual sovereignty, offering protection against negative influences and fostering spiritual growth.

Participating in Collective Rituals: Collective rituals, such as group meditation, Havan, and Kirtan (devotional singing), amplify the spiritual energy generated by each participant. These rituals create a powerful environment of protection and purification, enhancing the spiritual sovereignty of all who take part. Participating in collective rituals helps to reinforce individual practices, creating a strong, unified field of spiritual energy that guards against parasitic influences.

EMBRACING A HOLISTIC APPROACH TO SPIRITUAL SOVEREIGNTY

Integrating Body, Mind, and Spirit: Hindu practices emphasize the importance of addressing the whole being—body, mind, and spirit—in the pursuit of spiritual sovereignty. This holistic approach ensures that all aspects of the individual are aligned and protected. By integrating physical purification, mental discipline, and spiritual devotion, individuals can create a strong, resilient foundation that supports their spiritual sovereignty.

Living in Harmony with Nature: Hinduism teaches that living in harmony with nature is essential for maintaining spiritual sovereignty. This includes following a sattvik diet, engaging in regular detoxification practices, and honoring the cycles of nature through rituals and observances. By living in alignment with natural principles, individuals can protect themselves from parasitic influences and cultivate a deep, abiding connection to the divine.

Reclaiming and maintaining spiritual sovereignty is a sacred journey that requires dedication, mindfulness, and the integration of ancient wisdom into modern life. Hindu practices, with their rich tradition of rituals, mantras, and meditations, offer powerful tools for protecting the spirit, purifying the body and mind, and strengthening the connection to the divine.

By embracing these practices, individuals can create a protective shield against negative influences, including parasitic forces, and cultivate a state of spiritual clarity and strength. The power of mantras, the transformative potential of rituals, and the discipline of regular spiritual practice all contribute to a holistic approach to spiritual sovereignty that honors the interconnectedness of body, mind, and spirit.

As you continue on this journey, remember that spiritual sovereignty is not a destination but an ongoing process of growth, purification, and connection. By integrating these ancient practices into your daily life, you can protect yourself from the challenges of modern life and cultivate a state of health, well-being, and spiritual fulfillment that supports your highest potential.

In today's fast-paced world, the ancient wisdom of Ayurveda and Hinduism offers timeless guidance for maintaining physical health, mental clarity, and spiritual sovereignty. However, integrating these practices into modern life can be challenging due to the demands of work, family, and social responsibilities. This chapter provides practical advice on how to incorporate Ayurvedic and Hindu principles into daily life, focusing on diet, detoxification, spiritual practices, and lifestyle choices that support holistic well-being and minimize exposure to parasitic influences. It also encourages a cultural shift away from meat consumption, promoting a Sattvik lifestyle that aligns with both ancient wisdom and contemporary needs.

INTEGRATING AYURVEDA AND HINDUISM IN MODERN LIFE

DAILY PRACTICES FOR HEALTH AND SPIRITUALITY

The foundation of a healthy and spiritually sovereign life lies in daily practices that nurture the body, mind, and spirit. Ayurveda and Hinduism offer a wealth of practices that can be easily integrated into daily routines, providing a holistic approach to health that addresses all aspects of the individual.

MAINTAINING STRONG DIGESTIVE FIRE (AGNI)

Dietary Choices: In Ayurveda, maintaining a strong digestive fire (Agni) is essential for overall health and well-being. A balanced diet that includes fresh, whole foods, and avoids processed, heavy, or tamasic foods is key to supporting Agni. Eating at regular intervals, avoiding overeating, and consuming foods that are easy to digest help to keep the digestive fire burning brightly, which in turn supports the body's ability to resist parasitic infections and maintain overall health.

Mindful Eating: Mindful eating is a practice that involves paying full attention to the act of eating, savoring each bite, and being aware of the body's hunger and satiety signals. By eating mindfully, individuals can enhance digestion, reduce stress, and prevent overeating, all of which contribute to maintaining a strong Agni. Mindful eating also fosters a deeper connection with the food being consumed, recognizing it as a source of nourishment for both body and spirit.

Herbs and Spices: Incorporating Ayurvedic herbs and spices into daily meals can help to support digestion and protect against parasites. Spices such as ginger, cumin, turmeric, and coriander are known for their digestive and anti-parasitic properties. Regular use of these spices in cooking not only enhances the flavor of food but also promotes digestive health and resilience against infections.

PRACTICING REGULAR DETOXIFICATION

Seasonal Cleansing: Ayurveda emphasizes the importance of regular detoxification, particularly during the transition between seasons. Seasonal cleansing helps to remove accumulated toxins (Ama) from the body, prevent disease, and maintain balance in the doshas. Practices such as fasting, Panchakarma, and herbal cleanses can be incorporated into seasonal routines to support **detoxification and rejuvenation.**

Daily Detoxification Rituals: In addition to seasonal cleansing, daily detoxification rituals can be easily integrated into modern life. Practices such as oil pulling, dry brushing, tongue scraping, and drinking warm water with lemon in the morning help to support the body's natural detoxification processes. These simple practices can be performed as part of a daily routine, providing ongoing support for digestion, detoxification, and overall health.

Hydration and Cleansing: Staying well-hydrated is essential for detoxification and overall health. Drinking sufficient water throughout the day helps to flush out toxins, support digestion, and maintain healthy skin and organs. Herbal teas, such as those made from ginger, fennel, or mint, can also support digestion and detoxification, providing additional benefits beyond hydration.

ADHERING TO A SATTVIK LIFESTYLE

Sattvik Diet: A Sattvik diet, which emphasizes purity, balance, and lightness, is central to maintaining physical and spiritual health. This diet is predominantly vegetarian, focusing on fresh fruits, vegetables, whole grains, legumes, nuts, and seeds. It avoids meat, processed foods, excessive spices, and stimulants, all of which can disturb the mind and body. By following a Sattvik diet, individuals can maintain a strong digestive fire, reduce the risk of parasitic infections, and support mental and spiritual clarity.

Cleanliness and Hygiene: Cleanliness is an important aspect of the Sattvik lifestyle, both in terms of personal hygiene and the environment. Regular bathing, washing hands before meals, and maintaining a clean living space help to prevent the accumulation of toxins and parasites. This emphasis on cleanliness extends to the preparation and consumption of food, where fresh, clean ingredients are used to nourish the body and spirit.

Moderation and Balance: The Sattvik lifestyle promotes moderation in all aspects of life, including diet, sleep, work, and recreation. By avoiding extremes and maintaining balance, individuals can reduce stress, prevent disease, and maintain spiritual sovereignty. This balanced approach to life supports physical health, mental clarity, and spiritual well-being.

THE CULTURAL SHIFT: MOVING BEYOND MEAT CONSUMPTION

One of the most significant cultural shifts that can enhance health and spiritual sovereignty is the move away from meat consumption. In both Ayurveda and Hinduism, meat is considered tamasic—meaning it is heavy, impure, and can dull the mind and spirit. Reducing or eliminating meat from the diet can have profound effects on physical, mental, and spiritual health, as well as on the environment and society.

THE IMPACT OF MEAT ON HEALTH AND SPIRITUALITY

Physical Health: Meat, particularly red meat, is difficult to digest and can create Ama (toxins) in the body. It is also a significant source of parasitic infections, as many parasites are transmitted through the consumption of undercooked or contaminated meat. By reducing or eliminating meat from the diet, individuals can improve digestion, reduce the risk of parasitic infections, and promote overall health.

Mental and Spiritual Clarity: In Ayurveda and Hinduism, meat is believed to have a tamasic quality, meaning it can dull the mind, reduce mental clarity, and disconnect individuals from their spiritual path. Consuming a vegetarian or Sattvik diet, on the other hand, is believed to enhance mental clarity, support spiritual practices, and promote a deeper connection with the divine.

Karmic and Ethical Considerations: Hinduism teaches that all living beings are interconnected and that harming another creature creates negative karma. By choosing a vegetarian diet, individuals align themselves with the principle of Ahimsa (non-violence), reducing harm to other beings and generating positive karma. This alignment with ethical and spiritual principles further strengthens spiritual sovereignty and promotes a sense of peace and harmony.

ENCOURAGING A PLANT-BASED DIET

Practical Tips for Transitioning: Transitioning to a plant-based diet can be challenging, especially for those accustomed to a meat-centric diet. Start by gradually reducing meat consumption, perhaps beginning with one or two meatless days per week. Experiment with plant-based recipes that are satisfying and nutritious, and explore new ingredients and cooking techniques to keep meals interesting and enjoyable.

Nutritional Considerations: A well-planned vegetarian or plant-based diet can provide all the nutrients needed for optimal health. Ensure that meals include a variety of fruits, vegetables, whole grains, legumes, nuts, and seeds to provide a balance of protein, fiber, vitamins, and minerals. If needed, consider supplementing with vitamin B12, iron, and omega-3 fatty acids, which can be more challenging to obtain from a vegetarian diet.

The Sattvik Diet in Modern Life: The principles of the Sattvik diet can be easily adapted to modern life, even in busy or demanding schedules. Plan meals ahead of time, keep a well-stocked pantry of healthy staples, and make use of simple, quick recipes that emphasize fresh, whole foods. By incorporating Sattvik principles into daily meals, individuals can enjoy the benefits of a clean, nourishing diet that supports both physical and spiritual health.

PROMOTING A CULTURAL SHIFT

Advocating for Change: Promoting a cultural shift away from meat consumption requires both individual action and collective advocacy. Share the benefits of a plant-based or Sattvik diet with friends, family, and community members, and encourage others to explore these dietary choices. Support local initiatives and organizations that promote vegetarianism, sustainable agriculture, and ethical food practices.

Education and Awareness: Education is key to promoting a cultural shift in dietary habits. Provide resources, information, and guidance on the health, environmental, and spiritual benefits of a plant-based diet. Host workshops, cooking classes, or discussions that explore the principles of Ayurveda, the Sattvik lifestyle, and the impact of food choices on health and well-being.

Leading by Example: One of the most powerful ways to promote change is by leading by example. By embodying the principles of the Sattvik lifestyle and demonstrating the benefits of a plant-based diet, individuals can inspire others to make similar choices. Whether through personal interactions, social media, or community involvement, leading by example can have a ripple effect that encourages a broader cultural shift toward health, sustainability, and spiritual sovereignty.

INTEGRATING SPIRITUAL PRACTICES IN DAILY LIFE

In addition to dietary and lifestyle choices, integrating spiritual practices into daily life is essential for maintaining spiritual sovereignty and overall well-being. Hinduism offers a wide range of practices that can be adapted to modern life, providing tools for spiritual growth, protection, and connection.

DAILY RITUALS AND PRACTICES

Morning Rituals: Begin each day with a morning ritual that sets a positive tone for the day. This can include simple practices such as lighting a candle or incense, offering a prayer or mantra, and spending a few moments in meditation or contemplation. Morning rituals help to center the mind, connect with the divine, and create a sense of purpose and direction for the day ahead.

Evening Rituals: Just as morning rituals help to start the day with intention, evening rituals provide an opportunity to reflect on the day, release stress, and prepare for restful sleep. Practices such as journaling, chanting, or performing Aarti (offering light) can help to clear the mind, calm the emotions, and cultivate gratitude and peace before bed.

Mindfulness Throughout the Day: Incorporating mindfulness into daily activities helps to maintain spiritual awareness and presence. Whether eating, working, or interacting with others, approach each activity with mindfulness and intention. This practice of mindfulness helps to keep the mind focused, reduce stress, and maintain a connection with the present moment.

INCORPORATING MEDITATION AND MANTRA PRACTICES

Daily Meditation: Meditation is a cornerstone of spiritual practice in Hinduism, offering a way to quiet the mind, deepen spiritual awareness, and connect with the divine. Set aside time each day for meditation, whether it is a few minutes or longer. Choose a meditation technique that resonates with you, such as focusing on the breath, visualizing a deity, or repeating a mantra.

Mantra Repetition: Mantras are powerful tools for spiritual protection and growth. Incorporate mantra repetition (Japa) into your daily routine, using a mala (prayer beads) to keep count. Whether reciting the Mahamrityunjaya Mantra for protection, the Gayatri Mantra for clarity, or a personal mantra, this practice helps to align the mind with divine energy and create a protective shield against negativity.

Group Meditation and Chanting: Participating in group meditation or chanting sessions, either in person or online, can amplify the benefits of individual practice. The collective energy generated in group settings enhances the vibrational impact of the practice, creating a powerful environment for spiritual growth and protection.

INTEGRATING RITUALS INTO MODERN LIFE

Adapting Rituals to Contemporary Life: Traditional Hindu rituals can be adapted to fit the demands of modern life. Simplify rituals where necessary, focusing on the intention and essence of the practice rather than the details. For example, if performing a full Puja (worship ceremony) is not feasible, consider lighting a candle, offering a simple prayer, or chanting a mantra as a way to maintain a connection with the divine.

Incorporating Rituals into Family Life: Involve family members in spiritual rituals, creating a shared practice that strengthens bonds and fosters spiritual growth. Family rituals, such as performing Aarti together, reciting a mantra before meals, or celebrating festivals with traditional practices, help to create a spiritual foundation for the entire household.

Creating Sacred Spaces: Designate a space in your home for spiritual practice, where you can perform rituals, meditate, or simply spend time in contemplation. This sacred space serves as a reminder of the importance of spiritual practice and provides a peaceful environment for connecting with the divine.

THE PATH FORWARD: EMBRACING A HOLISTIC APPROACH

Integrating Ayurveda and Hinduism into modern life requires a holistic approach that addresses the physical, mental, and spiritual aspects of well-being. By adopting a Sattvik lifestyle, practicing regular detoxification, and incorporating daily spiritual practices, individuals can maintain health, protect against parasitic influences, and cultivate spiritual sovereignty.

ALIGNING WITH NATURE

Living in Harmony with Natural Rhythms: Ayurveda and Hinduism both emphasize the importance of living in harmony with natural rhythms, such as the cycles of the seasons, the phases of the moon, and the daily rising and setting of the sun. Aligning with these rhythms supports physical health, mental clarity, and spiritual connection. Incorporate practices such as seasonal detoxification, lunar observances, and daily rituals that honor the natural cycles.

Embracing Sustainability: Living in harmony with nature also means embracing sustainable practices that protect the environment and promote long-term well-being. Choose eco-friendly products, reduce waste, and support sustainable agriculture. By making choices that respect the earth and its resources, individuals contribute to the health of the planet and align themselves with the principles of Ayurveda and Hinduism.

CULTIVATING MINDFULNESS AND PRESENCE

Mindfulness in Action: Mindfulness is a key aspect of both Ayurveda and Hinduism, promoting awareness and presence in every moment. Practice mindfulness in daily activities, such as eating, working, and interacting with others. By staying present and aware, individuals can reduce stress, enhance mental clarity, and deepen their spiritual connection.

Mindfulness in Relationships: Cultivating mindfulness in relationships helps to create harmony and understanding. Approach interactions with others with kindness, patience, and empathy, recognizing the divine presence in each person. Mindful communication and active listening strengthen relationships and support a peaceful, balanced life.

EMBRACING CONTINUOUS LEARNING AND GROWTH

Lifelong Learning: The journey of integrating Ayurveda and Hinduism into modern life is one of continuous learning and growth. Seek out opportunities to expand your knowledge of these traditions, whether through books, classes, or personal study. Embrace the process of learning as a lifelong practice that deepens understanding and enhances spiritual growth.

Personal Reflection and Self-Study: Regular self-reflection and Svadhyaya (self-study) are important aspects of spiritual growth. Take time to reflect on your spiritual practices, lifestyle choices, and personal growth. Use journaling, meditation, or discussion with a spiritual mentor to explore your experiences, challenges, and progress on the path of integrating Ayurveda and Hinduism into your life.

Integrating the ancient wisdom of Ayurveda and Hinduism into modern life offers a path to holistic well-being, spiritual sovereignty, and alignment with the natural world. By embracing a Sattvik lifestyle, practicing regular detoxification, and incorporating daily spiritual practices, individuals can protect themselves from parasitic influences, maintain physical and mental health, and cultivate a deep connection with the divine.

This journey of integration is not a one-time event but an ongoing process of learning, growth, and adaptation. It requires mindfulness, dedication, and a commitment to living in harmony with the principles of Ayurveda and Hinduism. As individuals make these practices a part of their daily lives, they not only enhance their own well-being but also contribute to a broader cultural shift toward health, sustainability, and spiritual sovereignty.

CONCLUSION:

THE PATH TO LIBERATION

As we conclude this exploration of the ancient wisdom of Ayurveda and Hinduism, it becomes clear that the path to health, spiritual sovereignty, and liberation is a holistic one. The interconnectedness of body, mind, and spirit is a central theme in these traditions, and it is through the integration of their teachings that we can reclaim control over our lives, resist the influence of parasitic forces, and cultivate a deep connection with the divine.

THE PATH TO LIBERATION

SYNTHESIS OF AYURVEDIC AND HINDU WISDOM

Throughout this book, we have delved into the profound insights offered by Ayurveda and Hinduism on the nature of parasites, both physical and spiritual. We have explored how these ancient traditions provide a comprehensive framework for understanding and addressing the threats posed by parasitic influences, not just as biological entities, but as forces that can undermine our mental clarity, spiritual sovereignty, and overall well-being.

THE INTERCONNECTEDNESS OF BODY, MIND, AND SPIRIT

Holistic Health: Ayurveda teaches that true health is not merely the absence of disease but a state of complete physical, mental, and spiritual well-being. This holistic approach recognizes that the body, mind, and spirit are deeply interconnected, and that imbalances in one aspect can affect the others. By maintaining balance through diet, detoxification, and spiritual practices, we can protect ourselves from parasitic influences and achieve a state of harmony and health.

Spiritual Sovereignty: Hinduism emphasizes the importance of spiritual sovereignty—the ability to maintain control over one's own mind, body, and spirit in the face of external influences. This sovereignty is achieved through regular spiritual practices, such as meditation, mantra chanting, and rituals, which fortify the individual's connection to the divine and create a protective barrier against negative forces. By embracing these practices, we can reclaim our autonomy and resist the subtle yet pervasive influences that seek to undermine our spiritual path.

THE ROLE OF FASTING AND THE SATTVIK LIFESTYLE

Fasting as a Spiritual Discipline: Fasting has been shown to be a powerful tool for both physical detoxification and spiritual purification. In Hinduism, fasting is not merely an act of abstaining from food, but a means of deepening one's connection to the divine and purifying the mind and body. This practice, which has been diminished or removed in other traditions, remains central in Hinduism, providing a means of maintaining spiritual clarity and resisting parasitic influences.

The Sattvik Lifestyle: The Sattvik lifestyle, with its emphasis on purity, balance, and simplicity, offers a blueprint for living in harmony with nature and maintaining health on all levels. By adopting a Sattvik diet, practicing regular detoxification, and embracing spiritual practices, we create an environment that is inhospitable to parasites and conducive to spiritual growth. This lifestyle not only supports physical health but also nurtures the mind and spirit, fostering a sense of peace, clarity, and connection with the divine.

THE CULTURAL AND ETHICAL DIMENSIONS OF DIET

Beyond Meat Consumption: One of the most significant insights offered by this exploration is the impact of meat consumption on both physical and spiritual health. Meat, particularly in its modern, industrialized form, is a major source of parasitic infections and is considered tamasic in Ayurveda, meaning it can dull the mind and spirit. By reducing or eliminating meat from our diets, we can not only protect ourselves from parasites but also align our lives with the ethical principles of non-violence (Ahimsa) and compassion for all beings.

Promoting a Plant-Based Future: The shift toward a plant-based diet is more than just a personal health choice; it is a cultural movement that has profound implications for the environment, society, and spiritual well-being. By embracing a vegetarian or Sattvik diet, we contribute to the sustainability of the planet, reduce harm to animals, and support a way of life that is in harmony with the principles of Ayurveda and Hinduism. This shift is a powerful step toward reclaiming spiritual sovereignty and creating a more compassionate and sustainable world.

A CALL TO ACTION: EMBRACE THE PATH TO LIBERATION

As we conclude this journey, it is important to recognize that the path to liberation—liberation from physical and spiritual parasites, from the influences that seek to control our minds and bodies, and from the cycles of ignorance and suffering—is one that requires conscious effort, dedication, and mindfulness. The wisdom of Ayurveda and Hinduism provides us with the tools we need to walk this path, but it is up to each of us to take the steps necessary to integrate these teachings into our lives.

1. TAKING PROACTIVE STEPS

Commit to Daily Practice: The first step in reclaiming spiritual sovereignty is to commit to a daily practice that nurtures the body, mind, and spirit. Whether it is through meditation, mantra chanting, fasting, or following a Sattvik diet, make a commitment to incorporate these practices into your daily routine. Consistency is key, and even small, daily actions can have a profound impact on your overall well-being.

Educate and Advocate: Share the insights you have gained from this exploration with others. Educate friends, family, and community members about the benefits of a plant-based diet, the importance of regular detoxification, and the power of spiritual practices in maintaining health and spiritual sovereignty. Advocate for changes in your community, whether it is through promoting vegetarianism, supporting sustainable agriculture, or encouraging spiritual practices that align with these ancient teachings.

2. CULTIVATING MINDFULNESS AND AWARENESS

Be Mindful of Your Choices: Every choice we make—what we eat, how we spend our time, the thoughts we cultivate—has an impact on our physical and spiritual health. Cultivate mindfulness in all aspects of your life, making choices that support your well-being and align with the principles of Ayurveda and Hinduism. By being mindful of your actions, you can reduce the influence of negative forces and create a life that is in harmony with your highest values.

Stay Connected to the Divine: Spiritual sovereignty is ultimately about maintaining a deep and abiding connection with the divine. Make time each day to nurture this connection, whether through prayer, meditation, or simply spending time in nature. This connection is the source of true strength and protection, and it is through this connection that we can find the guidance, support, and wisdom we need to navigate the challenges of life.

3. EMBRACING CONTINUOUS GROWTH

Learn and Grow: The journey to spiritual sovereignty and holistic health is an ongoing process of learning, growth, and self-discovery. Continue to explore the teachings of Ayurveda and Hinduism, deepen your spiritual practices, and remain open to new insights and experiences. This path is not static; it evolves as you evolve, and each step you take brings you closer to liberation and self-realization.

Adapt and Evolve: As you integrate these teachings into your life, be willing to adapt and evolve your practices to meet your changing needs and circumstances. Life is dynamic, and so too should be your approach to health and spirituality. Stay attuned to your body, mind, and spirit, and make adjustments as needed to maintain balance and harmony.

FINAL REFLECTIONS

The wisdom of Ayurveda and Hinduism offers a profound and comprehensive approach to health, spirituality, and liberation. By embracing these teachings, we can reclaim control over our lives, resist the influence of parasitic forces, and cultivate a deep connection with the divine. This journey is not without its challenges, but it is one that offers immense rewards—health, peace, clarity, and the freedom to live in alignment with our highest values.

As you move forward, may you find strength in the ancient wisdom that has guided countless generations, and may you walk the path to liberation with courage, compassion, and unwavering commitment to your own well-being and spiritual growth. The tools are in your hands; the journey is yours to undertake. May your path be blessed with light, love, and the protection of the divine.

With deep respect and guidance,

Dr. Sunayana Pandé

Dr. Sunayana Pandé, often referred to as Dr. Sun, is a multifaceted scholar, healer, and spiritual guide. With a profound academic background that includes multiple higher degrees in psychology, neuroscience, religion, and metaphysics, Dr. Sun combines rigorous scientific knowledge with deep spiritual wisdom to offer transformative guidance to individuals and communities.

ABOUT THE AUTHOR

Born into a Brahmin Hindu family with an impressive lineage from the foot of the Himalayas, Dr. Sun's early life was shaped by both the richness of her cultural heritage and the challenges of growing up in an abusive environment. These experiences profoundly influenced her work, leading her to develop innovative paradigms in mental health, spirituality, and wellness.

Dr. Sun is the founder of the Ardhanarishwara Temple, a sanctuary for non-binary persons, transgender individuals, and drag performers, established in response to oppressive legislation. This temple serves as a spiritual and community hub, offering a space for marginalized groups to explore their identities and find healing.

As a naturopathic doctor, metaphysician, therapist, and transformational coach, Dr. Sun's work is rooted in a holistic approach that addresses the mind, body, and spirit. She is particularly known for her groundbreaking work in developing a new paradigm for autism, which redefines the condition as a state of expanded consciousness rather than a disorder. This perspective is part of her broader commitment to neurodiversity and the acceptance of alternative states of consciousness.

Dr. Sun is also a prolific author, with several books to her name, including *Life in the Bliss Lane: Guide to Wellness, Self-Love, and Joy, Beyond Binary: Exploring Gender and Sexuality, You Make Me Sick: Virtue Signaling & Narcissistic Abuse, Pharmajuana: Guide to Cannabis for Cancer, Hidden Branches in the Family Tree: Navigating the NPE Experience, Why Straight Lines Don't Exist: Exploring Geometric Truths,* and *Bracing for Impact*, her memoir that explores her healing journey from familial abuse.

In her teaching and writing, Dr. Sunayana Pandé emphasizes the importance of self-compassion, forgiveness, and the integration of spiritual practices into daily life. Her courses, such as *The Pineal Portal: Turn Your Magic On* and *Quantum Vibration Mastery*, draw on cutting-edge research in neuroscience and metaphysics, combined with ancient wisdom from traditions like Hinduism and Rosicrucianism.

Through her work, Dr. Sun continues to inspire and lead with a message of inclusivity, compassion, and the power of the human spirit to overcome adversity and thrive. Her approach is progressive, liberal, and deeply rooted in the belief that healing and transformation are possible for everyone, regardless of their circumstances.

www.ingramcontent.com/pod-product-compliance
Lightning Source LLC
Chambersburg PA
CBHW071057240526
45471CB00016B/1975